I0791834

I Believe in Life BEFORE Death!

Know What to Do, How to Do It and Why You Do It.

Ronny Håkerud

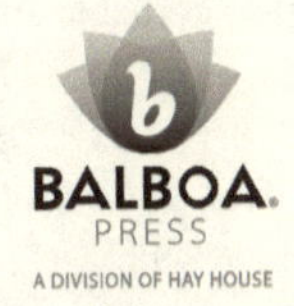

BALBOA. PRESS

A DIVISION OF HAY HOUSE

Balboa Press books may be ordered through booksellers or by contacting:

Balboa Press
A Division of Hay House
1663 Liberty Drive
Bloomington, IN 47403
www.balboapress.com
1 (877) 407-4847

Print information available on the last page.

ISBN: 978-1-9822-1708-2 (sc)
ISBN: 978-1-9822-1707-5 (hc)
ISBN: 978-1-9822-1715-0 (e)

Library of Congress Control Number: 2018914043

Balboa Press rev. date: 02/13/2019

Contents

Acknowledgments

To my wonderful wife, Anett, who has always been there for me, thank you for always taking such good care of our family. Thank you for being my loving wife. Without your support, this book would not been possible.

I would also like to thank my super-cool daughter Sofie for bringing inspiration, joy and hope to my life. You are my rock-star! You make the world a better place.

Thank you to all of you who have inspired me and challenged me in the search for a better understanding of our magnificent bodies and minds.

Thank you to all my patients, who trust me in taking care of the most important aspect of life, their health.

Thank you to you, my reader; may this book bring inspiration and action toward a long and fulfilling life.

Preface

I believe in life *before* death!

I want my life to be read like a good story—a story that is eventful. I want my life to be so much more than just survival. I will not feel cheated on my deathbed and think, *Is this all there is?* I would hope you feel the same. I would also like to be the author of my own story. This is the exact opposite of being a victim, who must live a live authored by others.

Through more than twenty years of health-related education, both formal and separate studies, and close to 100,000 patient consultations, I have come to understand how essential quality of life is. I would like to be a healthy and vital version of myself with a robust physique and condition, prepared to meet the challenges of today. I wish the same for my family, friends, patients, and for you. I want to use my skills and knowledge to help more people achieve these wishes and desires and to obtain the lives they deserve. Hopefully, you are one of them.

I was raised in a traditional family. While I was living at home with my family in the '70s and '80s, we followed the national recommendations. If someone had asked me twenty years ago about our way of life, I would without hesitation have said that my family had a healthy lifestyle. We were vaccinated. We were quickly taken to the doctor if anyone was feeling ill. The threshold for taking prescribed medications or over-the-counter medications was low.

Our diet was based on the traditional nationally sponsored food pyramid, with lots of carbohydrates and starches but little fats. Margarine was preferred in favor of real butter. "Light" products were common. For breakfast, I had cereals (for example, Corn Flakes) with pasteurized and homogenized cow's milk, often accompanied by a glass of milk. After my workouts, I often drank more than half a liter of cow's milk. We believed cow's milk was supposed to be important for our bone health. All fruits were healthy, and I could have as much as I wanted, anytime. I also remember I was very fond of eggs. Family friends of ours ran a hen farm. We bought lots of eggs from them—until the national recommendations advised us it was bad for our cholesterol level and could lead to heart attack, stroke, and clotted blood vessels. Once in my lifetime, I have had cavities. It was taken for granted that all four of my cavities were filled with amalgam. To keep my teeth healthy, I took fluor tablets every night after brushing my teeth with toothpaste filled with fluor. I thought the fluor tablets tasted nice.

Overall, my family did not question any of the national recommendations but, rather, followed them conscientiously.

I have had lots of health-related "aha" experiences on my health-related journey over the last twenty-five years. I had my first experiences when I studied philosophy and psychology during the '90s. I found it interesting to hear about the different views about who we are, the perennial questions, and especially about the mind-body relationship. I had never paid any conscious attention to these questions before. At the time, I started to realize that perhaps the truth I had been presented my whole life was not true at all.

My journey went on, first through studies in physical therapy and later in chiropractic and separate studies. I often asked myself, *Why has no one told me this before?* Often I have felt cheated, not by my parents, who conscientiously followed the national recommendations, but by the national recommendations themselves.

As a chiropractor I often meet people who come to me as a last resort. They say they have tried "everything." Of course, they get happy if I can help them, but often I find them frustrated and irritated at the same time. They say the same thing I used to say, "Why has no one told me that chiropractic could help for this particular problem?"

No one likes to be fooled or left out.

There are two simple steps to achieve well-being:

1. You have to find out what is good for you and what is bad for you.
2. You have to do what is good for you and avoid what is bad for you.

Why do so many fail if it is so easy? There are two major reasons:

1. You do not have the right information.
2. You have the right information, but you are in denial.

Through this book, I will elaborate thoroughly on these aspects.

Statistics show that we grow older and older, but I question the content in many people's lives. Yes, we are getting better at preventing early death and at keeping people alive, but statistically, we are not getting better at preventing sickness and disease, especially among the adults and elderly. While lifespan is one marker of health, so too is the quality of one's life.

Medical intervention can extend life expectancy, but is that our ultimate goal? When someone says they would love to live until they are eighty, ninety, or even a hundred, I think they say this because they envision a long life as an extension of the way they currently are living—not because they want to beat the statistics or just to exist.

We are all going to die, sooner or later. From my experience with thousands of patients, death is not our top concern. I believe losing the lifestyle that makes us happy is what concerns us more. It does not need to be a life-threatening disease. It could just as well be a disabling back, knee, or hip issue. We would like to continue to play tennis and feel the excitement of trying to beat our neighbor, continue to play golf in beautiful surroundings and try to get an even better handicap, continue to play soccer with our grandkids in the garden or be an affectionate spectator when our grandkids are scoring their first goal. We will continue to enjoy the quietness in the mountains as we hike through the spectacular scenery by foot or maybe by cross-country skiing. We will continue to feel the wind sweeping through our hair and the spray from the sea in our face while we are sailing. We will continue to travel to new destinations and explore the infinite possibilities. We will continue to tend our garden; to enjoy the scent from our beautiful flowers; and to reap our homegrown vegetables, berries, and fruits. We will continue to enjoy a tasteful meal in delightful company with family and friends. We would love to still be a valuable participant in society and an active friend and a loving and present family member. For me, these are examples of things I would like to be parts of my story.

If you read a good novel of any kind, I am pretty sure that you wonder how it ends. You are excited because you put effort into getting to know the different characters and vividly make pictures about the plot in your head. Do you think the ending would matter to you if you had only read the ending, without getting to know the characters or the plot? It is all the pages prior to the last chapter that makes the last chapter worth reading. Are you able to see a parallel to your life?

It's not the years in your life that count; it's the life in your years!

You might think that safety is regarded as an important ingredient in life, especially for the elderly. Interviews and studies show the opposite. Even when people are in need of care, safety is not top priority. The answer is crystal clear—we want to live, not just be kept alive! That is a major difference.

I remember vividly a patient from my internship as a physiotherapist. I was working at a rehabilitation unit with patients who had gone through amputations. This patient was a man in his sixties who had lost his leg due to decreased circulation to his feet. He was a heavy smoker, always surrounded by a cloud of smoke. He was also a diabetic. His list of medications was like a parchment. Our job at the rehabilitation center was to help him take care of his stump, fitting his prosthesis and giving him functional exercises. The man was very depressed and did not want any prosthesis. He was not interested in moving around, just wanting to sit in his wheelchair with his cigarettes and hide within the cloud. The other leg had developed a nasty ulcer and was, at the time, also in danger of being lost. When the man was released from the hospital to go home, he was informed about the importance of movement, the importance of taking care of his diabetes, and the consequences of heavy smoking.

Unfortunately, the man was back to our rehabilitation unit before my internship was over—this time without the other leg as well. If possible, he looked even more depressed. He told us he did not want to live anymore. His life was empty—no more pages to add to his story. I was puzzled that he still smoked like a chimney after losing both of his legs. On several occasions, the man fell asleep with his cigarette. He got a couple of nasty burns from the embers. He was also a fire hazard for the rest of us at the unit. I remember I got angry with him; how could he still smoke after losing both his legs? How could he be so stupid?

Today I see it differently. This man had obviously ended up in this terrible situation, crippled by double amputations, due to bad lifestyle choices. The amputations extended his life but certainly didn't improve his quality of life—a life he did not want to take part in. His life ended several years before his legs were amputated. The help he needed got to him far too late—not to extend his lifetime, but to save his life. He should have had help and healthy advice far earlier before the situation got out of hand. He may not have ended up in this shape if it was not for bad choices.

What if the man had received adequate information about the importance of eating well, moving well, and thinking well when he was young? Would he have found himself in the same situation he was in when I met him? I guess the man didn't have the right information about the danger of smoking in his early years. Later in life, I think he must have gotten the warning, but he decided to live in denial.

While I was writing parts of *I Believe in Life* before *Death!* I spoke with the landlord of the apartment I was renting. He told me he'd had his knee replaced less than a year ago. Now, he could not bend his knee to more than ninety degrees. He struggled with daily activities, and just to get up from the floor was bothersome. Because of his poor condition, he told me he'd just recently had to sell his farm, which he loved spending time at. It had been a place of recreation, peace, and tranquility for his wife and himself for several years. Now he seemed depressed and fragile.

He went on to tell me that, when he confronted his surgeon, explaining that his knee was preventing him from enjoying his daily activities, he was told he should be happy; ninety degrees was supposedly quite good, and after all, he did not have pain anymore. The landlord told me he felt cheated. This was not what he'd expected at this stage of life.

I think these examples illustrate three major aspects of life. First, quality of life is far more important than quantity. A 2011 study showed that 31 percent are more concerned about dementia than both cancer and death itself.[1]

Second, as health professionals, we need to be better at communicating the expected outcome to the patient. When a patient undergoes one heavy treatment after the other, I think he or she pictures more years like those he or she has already lived. While the doctor might think one to five years more to live with an aggressive treatment, the patient might think fifteen to twenty years and almost with the same lifestyle as before. The reality is, lifestyle is on the decline in everyway. The loved ones will observe the person they once knew slowly fading away and struggling to survive, a mere shadow of the person he or she used to be. There is no correlation between expectation and outcome.

Third, poor lifestyle choices lead us toward sickness and disease that could have been prevented with better recommendations. Unfortunately, I think lots of the national recommendations today are based on outdated knowledge and often influenced by an economical agenda. The recommendations are not in the best interest of the public. We now understand that the recommendations have been incorrect for several years, and change and education is desperately needed.

I would like to rephrase the term "health care" and call it what it actually is, "sick care." Sick care is good if you are sick, but what we are actually doing today is practicing sick care on a healthy population. We will not get any healthier in the long run by treating more sick people. We will be a healthier population by making sure we live healthy lifestyles from the beginning and preventing sickness in the first place!

"Maintaining order rather than correcting disorder is the ultimate principle of wisdom. To cure disease after it has appeared is like digging a well when one feels thirsty" (Huangdi Neijing, second century BC).

By all means, I think it is important that we are taken well care of when we do get sick, but the goal should always be to use sick care as little as possible. However, I want to be clear—sick care has its place and can be lifesaving without question. There are many skillful doctors, nurses, surgeons, and other medical practitioners who are highly skilled and ready to take care of sick people when needed. The point is that it is much better and easier to be and stay healthy rather than to become healthy after you have become sick. Since most sickness and diseases and aches and pains are lifestyle related, you should make healthy choices to stay healthy.

There is a problem when we use methods developed for sick people on a healthy population. Imagine a person with fever, runny nose, headache, nausea, diarrhea, and alternating sweat and chills. Conventional medicine would probably call this influenza or some kind of virus. Treatment would probably be something like acetaminophen/paracetamol for the fever and headache, nasal spray for the runny nose, Imodium for the diarrhea, metoclopramide for the nausea, and broad spectrum antibiotics for a possible bacterial infection, everything to remove the symptoms. My question is, Is this person really sick or are the symptoms this person's immune system in action, trying to keep the body in balance? Will the medication contribute to make the person healthier? Or is it just making the person feel better?

From a holistic point of view, when the immune system activates, the body heats up to make the condition less viable for bacteria and virus. The reason we vomit or have diarrhea is because these are mechanisms our body uses to get rid of something that does not belong in the body. Increased production of mucus is a defense mechanism to stop unwanted particles entering the body when we breathe.

The medication we are prescribed when we are sick will only camouflage the symptoms (which the body needs as feedback) and ultimately leads the person further away from a natural immune response and better health.

Are we being misled with modern medical practices of treating only the symptoms? I have definitely been misled. I have been misled to live a lifestyle that isn't bringing out the best of me. I am sure I am still being misled, but I am also sure I am much more difficult to mislead today than I was twenty-five years ago.

In May 2016, there was an announcement on the national news of a research team in Norway who had discovered a medication for type 2 diabetes. As you may know, type 2 diabetes is a lifestyle-induced disease reaching epidemic proportion today. With this new medication, type 2 diabetics no longer needed to measure blood glucose levels or inject insulin to counter the damaging high glucose levels in the body. They could just take the medication and continue to live their lives as they had done in the past. No need for physical activity, no need to change their nutrition or any change in lifestyle was advocated. While monitoring blood glucose level is important, there is far more to health than just the blood glucose level. The lifestyle leading to the increased blood glucose level is the core problem, not the blood glucose itself.

Society today is rough. As they say, "Money talks; bullshit walks." Science is synonymous with uncontested truth. Net trolls abounds. Spice it up with evolutionary quotes like "survival of the fittest" and a philosophy based on genes controlling our destiny, and you have a very hard race to win. Do we have a chance? Is life all about surviving?

To be able to become the best version of yourself, to take advantage of your qualities and fulfill your wishes and desires, I think it is especially important to question some of your basic premises. Your life shall not be a fight against a ticking clock or survival of the fittest. There is a reason why you are here. You are unique. You are part of a bigger puzzle, where all the pieces are equally as important. You are born for wellness and personal success.

Every day, I try to figure out more of our amazing, fascinating, and most often well-functioning dance between our body and mind. In *I Believe in Life* before *Death!* I will share my experiences and thoughts acquired from my studies and from my patients. Hopefully, these experiences and thoughts will help to make your own story about yourself eventful, loveable, and healthy. At the end of this book, I hope you will have learned something you can apply to your life, and hopefully, it should be a story to recommend to others.

"For dust you are and to dust you shall return"

We are a part of an ecosystem. There is nothing in us we can't find in nature. The human body consists exclusively of degradable organic material when we are born.

There is nothing humanity has done to bring us further away from nature that has been beneficial in the long run. We are a part of the whole. "The whole is more than the sum of its parts" (definition of holism, metaphysics, Aristotle).

Think about all the natural and amazing processes from conception to birth. Sperm from the man meets an egg from the woman; the egg is fertilized; and, during nine months, the egg develops to a newborn child. Of course the child is not fully developed, but it has all that it takes to live a healthy and good life.

Unfortunately, medication and surgery have become an integral part of modern society. According to the Norwegian Institute for Public Health, two-thirds of the Norwegian population is taking prescribed drugs. What happened to us? How did humans survive earlier when we did not have medications? Is nature suddenly not good enough? Where, in a lifespan, do the basic premises for a healthy life change?

There are two reasons why you are not feeling well or functioning at an optimum level—either you are lacking something natural, or you have too much of something natural.

Let's take a look at a dying plant. Most of us will probably think the plant lacks water or maybe another natural ingredient. Why do we think differently when it comes to human beings? Today, many people think of medication as their first option when they do not feel well. *I need to go to the doctor*, is often their first thought.

To make a point, I have asked a few of my patients if they ever give their plants medication? They always look at me strangely and probably think I have completely lost it. Of course they have not given their plants medication.

"They are natural," they respond.

"And how about yourself?" is my response.

In his book *The Turning Point*, Fritjof Capra calls the tools of a mechanistic and medical practice the three R's—repair, remove, and replace.[2]

Do you think you are not feeling well because you lack medications in your body or have spare limbs or organs? Another important question to think about is this: If you had free and unlimited access to medication and surgery, would you be healthier?

Do you look at pain as your friend or as your enemy? What if you were offered a pill, guaranteed free from side effects, which made you pain-free for the rest of your life? Would you take it?

Let's say you took this pill and you happened to fall down the stairs and break your foot—no pain! You kept going. However, now the foot became swollen, and you slowly began to lose control over your foot and your balance—no pain! Would you still have taken the pill?

When you came home, you made dinner. Your phone rang. While you were talking on the phone, you leaned onto the stove. You did not realize that you just got a nasty burn before you smelled burned skin—no pain! Would you still take the pill?

Pain is your friend trying to tell you an important message you should take notice of. If you have an important message to tell your friend and your friend does not listen, what do you do? You will probably raise your voice or use stronger words. The same principle applies for the body. If you do not listen, the symptom will come back even louder.

Homeostasis could be defined as a system in which variables are regulated so that internal conditions remain stable and relatively constant. Examples of homeostasis include the regulation of temperature and the balance between acidity and alkalinity (pH). Human homeostasis is the process that maintains the stability of the human body's internal environment in response to changes in external conditions (*Wikipedia*).

The pharmacological industry pushes us further and further away from homeostasis by adding chemicals or artificial additives to the body. Christopher Kent DC, JD, once said, "We do not live in a republic or a democracy, we live in a pharmocracy."

The way I see it, health care is too often not about our health. It is sick care, with medications and surgery as the only tools in the toolbox.

D. D. Palmer, founder of chiropractic, once said, "One question was always uppermost in my mind in my search for the cause of disease. I desired to know why one person was ailing and his associate, eating at the same table, working in the same shop, at the same bench, was not. Why? What difference was there in the two persons that caused one to have pneumonia, catarrh, typhoid or rheumatism, while his partner, similarly situated, escaped? Why?"

Remember, a symptom is never a cause but a consequence of a cause. Symptom-based treatment is called allopathy. Treatment of a symptom, without addressing its cause, will most likely not end well.

A good doctor knows what to do. Better doctors know how they do it. And the best doctors know why they are doing it.

Why are we using all our effort to wipe the floor (symptom) when we have a leakage from the roof (cause)? It is time to fix the roof, in addition to wiping up the floor. It is time to evaluate our way of living.

The Great Paradox

Most people search for wellness in one form or another. To reach toward, wellness I think it is highly important to establish some basic premises.

When we are born, we are born perfect, with the best possibility to achieve a healthy and good life. We have all the tools needed for wellness. That is one of my basic premises.

Look at your life as a painting. You are the artist, and you have the exact same colors Michelangelo or da Vinci had. You can choose to paint a colorful painting full of love and joy, or you can choose to paint a battlefield in shades of gray.

Look at your life as a melody. You are the composer, and you have the same eight notes as Beethoven, Bach, or Mozart had.

Look at your life as poetry. You can make your story the way you would like with the exact same twenty-six letters Ibsen or Hemingway had.

In other words, you have all the tools necessary to make the life of your dreams.

Another of my basic premises is that the human body is a self-regulating organism trying to maintain homeostasis. You do not need to think about how to repair a broken bone or digest food. Your innate intelligence will take care of it.

When you have established your basic premises, it will be a lot easier to take appropriate action so you can achieve your goals and get the life you desire.

If you think about cause and effect, wellness will be an effect of who you are, not the cause of what you do. Contradictions in your basic premises will lead to destruction later in life.

Let's say you think human beings are made for sickness and disease, with deficiencies only medications from the pharmaceutical industry can make up for. Then fever, inflammations, regulation of cholesterol, blood pressure, and insulin are only actions from the body to lead us toward sickness and disease.

If this were the case, I would agree it is a smart move to overrule the auto-regulation of the body with medications.

On the other hand, if my basic premises are right, medications are a contradiction and will lead to destruction later in life. If I get a fever, my immune system has probably recognized something that is harmful to my body and is trying to make the environment bad for the intruders. If I choose to take an antipyretic drug, it will be contradictory to my basic premises and lead to destruction later in life. I will probably feel better for the moment, but I will also allow the unfortunate processes to continue.

The great paradox is that most people will say they are made for wellness with all the tools necessary to achieve it, but at the same time they choose actions based on sickness and disease.

"John" is eighty-two years old. He came to my clinic because of a lower back problem and a stiff neck. He told me that he was very satisfied with his GP and his internist. At the same time, he gave me his list of medications. He gave me the impression that he was proud of this list. It seemed like he viewed it as evidence of him being well taken care of. John took medications for high blood pressure, atrial fibrillation, high cholesterol, and type 2 diabetes. He had sleeping pills, painkillers, anti-inflammatory, and antiemetic medications when needed. He added to the story that he'd also had six to seven injections of cortisone in one of his shoulders. He praised the doctor for being very good. The injections had such a great result—at the time.

At the same time, he had to admit that the shoulder pain came back regularly. The doctor had told him that it was normal for a man his age.

When I examined John, there were several findings. An x-ray of his spine detected major misalignments, scoliosis, increased thoracic kyphosis, forward head carriage, and a reversed cervical curve. In addition, there were degenerative changes in almost his entire spine, especially in his lower back and neck and also moderate changes in both hip joints.

There was also sclerosis of his aorta detected on the x-ray. From my observation, John had a big and bloated belly, but his arms and legs were skinny and looked fragile. He had a bad slouched posture, lacked balance, and was breathing heavily.

I was wondering, Had John been misled by "sick care"? His state of health was not good at all, but still he felt he had been taken well care of. All of his symptoms were lifestyle-related. But as far as I know, he had not received any recommendations for leading a better lifestyle.

On the contrary, he had been told to take the medications and keep on with the same lifestyle.

Symptoms are feedback from the body to better maintain homeostasis. Medication, where the goal is to stop auto-regulation, is contradictory to my basic premises.

John is slightly older than the average life expectancy in Norway. Conventional medicine will probably claim he is a success, based on his age. However, I am not so sure. I wonder if John could have had a better quality of life with better lifestyle choices. In my opinion, it does not matter if John is part of an increased life expectancy if the content of his life is poor.

I would like to add to the story about John that his GP had told him to stay away from chiropractors. John had been told the doctor knew more than one hundred patients who had been paralyzed after manipulations (of course, a claim that was fear based, not based on facts). After being exposed to the scare tactics from his GP, John must have been either desperate or very brave, since he paid me a visit. I will also add to the story that John slept through the whole night after his first neck adjustment, and he still does months later. It had been years since he'd had a good night's sleep.

"Ellen" presented to me with hip problems. She was in her late fifties and was overweight. She told me her hip problem started after she started to exercise because she wanted to lose weight, so she visited her doctor. He told her to rest, move as little as possible, and take Voltaren, an anti-inflammatory drug, every eight hours until the pain was gone. The doctor also wanted to give her antidepressants because she was depressed.

Ellen came to me because she had been pushed to do so by her daughter. Her daughter disagreed with her mother's doctor on how to treat her hip problem.

My focus was, like the doctor's, to relieve the stress to the hip— but note, just for the hip itself, not her entire body. Here, the analogy about wiping up the floor after a leak from the roof applies. It is a good thing to wipe up the floor, but you have to fix the roof as well. To fix her roof, we started to increase her blood supply to her hip by getting her up on a bike, with minimal resistance and without any load from the body to the hip. I also advised her to swim (a non-weight-bearing activity) and do some easy strengthening exercises, still without loading her hip much. We also talked about the importance of proper nutrition and handling of stress. At the same time, dysfunctions (subluxations) were corrected. The next phase included rehabilitation to regain proper function.

How can it be that two similar diagnoses lead to such different strategies? It must be because our basic premises are different.

Bad lifestyle is killing us

In Western society, health care is always a hot topic for the politicians. But are they actually talking about health care? Or is it sick care? All focus goes toward how to put out a fire, or a symptom rather. There are little funds given to preventative health care. Isn't it quite sensational that we spend more and more money to put out fires, but more fires are created than ever before?

We are all going to die sooner or later. A few generations back, people died their "natural" deaths caused by old age, despite dying at a younger age than what is average today. Do you hear about anyone dying from old age today? We hear about heart disease, dementia, Parkinson's, diabetes, and so on. Today, most people die undergoing some kind of treatment.

Let us take a closer look at the most common causes of death today.

The number one cause of death is cardiovascular disease, which half of us will die from. Number two on the list is cancer. One out of three will get cancer. Number three on the list (depending on which studies you look at) is iatrogenic disease. This is damage or injury caused by medical interventions, such as medicine or surgery. Number four on the list is disease related to obesity.

The commonality of all of the above is that they are lifestyle-related diseases, including cancer, and might be a consequence of poor choices. Despite this widespread knowledge, most of "health care" funds go to the fire department to put out fires (medicine, surgery, hospital, stem-cell research, and so on), and little goes to prevention and maintenance (physical activity, handling of stress, nutrition, chiropractic, and so on).

Cardiovascular disease

Cardiovascular disease affects the heart or blood circulation in one way or another, resulting in hypertension (elevated blood pressure), atherosclerosis (plaque in the vessel wall), heart infarction or arrhythmia (abnormal heart rhythm). The heart is a big muscle pumping blood around in the body through its vessels. The main functions of the cardiovascular system are transportation of nutrients from the digestive system, transportation of oxygen from the respiratory system, and elimination of waste products and carbon dioxide to maintain homeostasis in the body.

When the cardiovascular system is working properly, you should be able to adapt to different challenges. Your heart will beat faster when you are exercising, and your blood pressure will increase to make sure your cells get the nutrients needed. You will also breath faster to get more oxygen to the cells. If you are cold, you will start to shiver, and your blood vessels to your skin, arms, and legs will constrict to be able to keep the central vital parts of your body warm. If you get injured, white blood cells will be called upon to fight infections and promote healing.

Do you think you are healthy if you are not in pain? Many do. Cardiovascular disease is a disease that has few symptoms and, for that reason, is a good example of a disease that can catch people unaware. The first symptom of cardiovascular disease could be death. The heart has most likely not been healthy for quite some time. You can be one day away from dying and still feel fine. My granddad did. Most of us know someone close who, unfortunately, has had this experience. You have probably also heard about examples in the media when elite athletes have had some kind of cardiac arrest in the prime of their athletic lives.

In most cases, cardiovascular disease is lifestyle related. Still, current interventions from conventional medicine are medications and surgery. Medications could be antihypertensive medicine, statins to lower cholesterol, or anticoagulants to prevent the blood from clotting. In 2013, 40 percent of the Norwegian population between seventy and seventy-nine years old took cholesterol-lowering medicine, while 70 percent of the population between eighty and eighty-nine years old took antihypertensive medicine. In

2014, 844, 336 Norwegians received a prescription for some kind of cardiovascular medicine. If we also include cholesterol-lowering medicine, the number is 1,362,670 people, which is more than one out of five inhabitants.[3]

How can it be that most of the people who die of cardiovascular disease take cardiovascular medication? To prescribe antihypertensive drugs for high blood pressure caused by an unhealthy lifestyle without mentioning lifestyle changes is, at best, misleading.

If you are in doubt about how your cardiovascular system works, you could do this simple test. First, measure your blood pressure or heart rate at rest. Then walk briskly up a few floors and measure your blood pressure or heart rate again. I guess you will find both your heart rate and your blood pressure is elevated. Can you think of the reason behind this reaction? Your muscle cells needs more nutrients to be able to perform the physical exercise. Your cardiovascular system responds by increasing your heart rate and your blood pressure. Did you notice that you got a more rapid breath as well? You will breathe more rapidly so that your blood cells can absorb more oxygen, which is another nutrient for your muscle cells.

If you live an active lifestyle, your blood pressure, heart rate, and breathing rate should vary through the entire day, trying to keep your body in homeostasis. You are healthy and adaptable.

To live with a constantly elevated blood pressure caused by a busy, stressful, and unhealthy lifestyle could be dangerous. Worst case, it can lead to a stroke and death. Most of the medical profession will most likely solve the problem by giving the person with elevated blood pressure antihypertensive drugs.

But let me ask you a question. What do you think will happen if you continue to live a busy, stressful, and unhealthy lifestyle demanding an elevated blood pressure and, at the same time, take antihypertensive medicine to lower your blood pressure to normal values? Do you think the problem is solved now? Your lifestyle is still the same. Wouldn't it be similar to watering your garden with a dripping garden hose? There will be no stress on the garden hose itself, but will your garden get enough water? Could a lack of lifestyle change be a cause of why most people who die from cardiovascular disease are taking medications for the same thing?

Another choice for the cardiovascular-diseased patient from conventional medicine is surgery. It could be a bypass surgery, where a clotted blood vessel to the heart will be replaced with a healthy blood vessel from the thigh to provide proper blood supply to the heart. It could also be blocking of clotted vessels or open-heart surgery to repair a heart valve. When the situation is out of control, these options are good and, in many cases, lifesaving. But at the same time, these options will never address the cause of the problem. It would have been so much better if we could have had a healthy lifestyle to prevent us from necessary sick care.

Cancer

With the occurrence and mortality of cancer today, about one-third of the Norwegian population will get cancer before turning seventy-five years old (the Norwegian Institute of Public Health). In many people's opinions, more people die from cancer in modern times than did in the past because of the unhealthy lifestyle adopted by industrialized countries.

A 2003 study, looked at the correlation between mortality from cancer and obesity.[4] The result showed obesity had an increased mortality rate from cancer. If you understand that glucose helps cancer cells to survive and that glucose is the foundation of many Western diets, these results are not very surprising.

Your body is made of trillions of cells. To keep your body healthy and in homeostasis, your cells will form, grow, divide, and die on a regular bases. They act like a well-functioning society, where different cells have their own unique function with an adapted cell cycle.

Sometimes, new cells, not needed, will form. Other times, old cells that are supposed to die and be replenished by new cells, will continue to live. When cells divide out of control, it is called cancer. This process happens every day. Your immune system should take care of it and keep your body in homeostasis. An analogy would be that you are producing garbage in your household. What will happen if your garbage is not removed? How long will it take before it gets uncomfortable? How long does it take before you get sick?

Poor lifestyle choices will weaken your body. It could be due to stress, toxins, lack of physical activity, or poor nutrition. Cancer cells will have a greater chance of developing if your body is weakened. Cancer will attack the weakest link. Some forms of cancer are genetically predisposed, but the major cause of cancer is related to an unhealthy lifestyle.[5]

Options of treatment for cancer are radiotherapy, chemotherapy, hormone therapy, and surgery, often combined. In the same way as the typical treatments for cardiovascular disease, these actions will not lead to fewer incidents of cancer. This is sick care and the fire department in action putting out fires. To be a more healthy society, we need more people who will not get sick.

"Illnesses hover constantly above us, their seeds blown by the wind, but they do not set in the terrain unless the terrain is ready to receive them" (Claude Barnard).[6]

Obesity

One of the leading health problems is obesity, which strikes the poor (who stuff themselves with hamburgers and pizza) even more severely than the rich (who eat organic salads and drink smoothies made of fruit). Each year, the US population spends more money on diets than the amount needed to feed all the hungry people in the rest of the world. Obesity is a double victory for consumerism. Instead of eating little, people eat too much, and then they buy diet products.

The World Health Organization issued a warning in 2016—obesity among children will be the greatest threat to our health in the future! In the report (*Ending Child Obesity*) the WHO urgently encourages all nations to take action and cooperate to meet this fast-growing problem.

The unrelenting global growth in obesity is not just confined to industrialized countries. It depends on the environment; if children grow up in unhealthy environments with poor nutrition, little physical activity, and too much time in front of a screen, they have a higher chance of being obese. In 2014, 41 million children were found to be obese (WHO). Obesity is not only a problem for our kids. More and more men and women fit the definition for obesity set by WHO.

A forty-year-old Norwegian is five kilograms heavier today than a forty-year-old in 1985. If we use the standards set by WHO, more than half of the Norwegian population between forty and forty-five years old is overweight today (the National Institute of Public Health).

With increasing weight there is an increased chance of type 2 diabetes; gall bladder disease; sleep apnea; cardiovascular disease; high blood pressure; degenerative changes in hips and knees; and some forms of cancer, like cancer of the colon among men (the National Institute of Public Health). In most cases, being overweight is lifestyle related, primarily lack of physical activity and poor nutrition. You can look at being overweight as a symptom. It tells you that you are not living a lifestyle optimal for your health. It is like the warning signs on the dashboard in your car. You can probably ignore the signs and pretend nothing has happened for a while. But when will the car break down? When will your body break down? Will you take the chance of continuing with the same lifestyle if you are overweight?

More than 8 percent of people with type 2 diabetes are overweight.[7]

Diabetes is a physical state of being where the body can't regulate the blood sugar level properly. The pancreas does not produce enough insulin to meet the need from the sugar intake. There are two types of diabetes, type 1 and type 2. Type 1 diabetes most often affects children and youth and is caused by a dysfunction of the pancreas—regardless of lifestyle. People with type 1 diabetes will benefit from a healthy lifestyle but will be dependent on insulin injection to keep the blood sugar level right. Just 10 percent of diabetics have type 1 diabetes.

Type 2 diabetes is different. It usually starts with a resistance to insulin brought on by a relentless supply of glucose over time. To compensate for the resistance, the pancreas needs to produce more insulin. The pancreas will eventually be overused and exhausted and not able to produce insulin at the same level anymore. Type 2 diabetes is mainly caused by bad lifestyle choices like lack of physical activity, being overweight, poor nutrition, and mental stress.[8]

All the organs in your body are highly dependent on a stable blood sugar level, especially your brain. A small change in blood sugar level can have a fatal outcome. There is about one teaspoon of sugar circulating in our blood at all times. If the level rises to one tablespoon, you will most likely die. In the United States, people consume about 75 mg of sugar every day on average.

A healthy lifestyle should not include more than about 15 mg of sugar intake on a daily basis. This is about the sugar level of a ripe mango. Insulin causes an increased cell division, which ultimately means we will also grow older faster. However, it also means it will increase the rate of division of cancer cells.

To lower blood sugar level, today's treatment will be insulin injections. This is a good option if the pancreas is dysfunctional. If the increased blood sugar level is caused by a previous and continuing unhealthy lifestyle, it will be a poor choice of treatment, as the lifestyle that causes type 2 diabetes will continue to degrade the body. More insulin will be a good choice for the pharmaceutical companies though.

Iatrogenic deaths

A study from medical clinics in the United States in 2006 registered 783,936 iatrogenic deaths per year. Iatrogenic means inflicted by medical staff in a form of treatment or surgery. To compare, a little less than 700,000 died from cardiovascular disease, and 550,000 from cancer.

These numbers were presented in "Death by Medicine," written by three medical doctors, one of them with a PhD in philosophy.[9]

According to the Journal of the American Medical Association, in 2000, 225,000 died from an iatrogenic cause in the United States.[10] [11] A study by Null et al. in 2003 looked into national statistics in the United States over a ten-year period and found iatrogenic deaths to be the top cause of people dying. More than 300,000 people died every year from an iatrogenic cause. This is equal to two jumbo jets packed with people every day, only in the United States. I doubt this information would stimulate more air traffic.

As a health care provider, my first commandment is "primum non nocere," which means "do no harm". It does not look like this commandment is valid for the pharmaceutical industry.

It is a great paradox that medical treatment is among the top three causes of death for human beings. I also find it alarming that all the deaths are justified by the cost of running a medical practice.

A meta-analysis published in the American Medical Association in 1998 reports that 2.2 million patients suffer from severe adverse reactions from prescribed medications. What is even more sensational is that 106,000 patients are dying from these adverse reactions.[12]

Money talks

Why is health less interesting than disease? Disease does not occur other than when the prerequisites for good health cease.

Unfortunately, I think the answer is partly economically related.

Health care, as it currently operates, will never lead to a healthier population as long as it is based on disease, as opposed to good health. We need more people who are less sick. Good health does not exist in a pill form, at the hospital, or under an operating knife. These measures are indications of an already bad lifestyle.

Preliminary calculations show that total health-related expenses in Norway were well over 288 billion kroner in 2013. This constitutes 9.6 percent of the gross domestic product and equals in excess of 56,700 kroner per resident.

Are we getting our "money's worth"? Measured in volume, health-related expenses have increased by around 20 percent in the last ten years.

It is not by way of chance that the pharmaceutical industry maintains the largest profit margin in the world. In a book written by Marcia Angell MD, who otherwise was the first female chief editor of the prestigious *New England Journal of Medicine*, writes that, in 2001, the largest pharmaceutical companies, who are included in Fortune 500, have on average a profit after taxes of 18.5 percent. In comparison, the other companies on the same list had an average profit of 3.3 percent. In 2002, the ten largest pharmaceutical companies in Fortune 500 earned more than the other 490 companies on the same list combined!

We must remember that most of the so-called "scientific" evidence behind recent medical practice is sponsored and paid for by these same pharmaceutical companies. Statistics from the United States show that pharmaceutical companies spend almost twice as much money on marketing as they spend on research and development of new medicine.[13] In 2004, Pfizer allocated almost US$120 million just for marketing purposes by Lipitor (cholesterol-lowering medication).

Although these pharmaceutical companies have high profit margins, they do everything they can to earn more. It is costly to develop, test, and market new medicine. We find "old" medicine constantly used in new areas. They can be used for completely different symptoms than the ones they were tested for. For example, I frequently hear about people who receive blood pressure medication or blood thinners for headaches, or young girls who get recommended the birth control pill for headaches or pimples.

Recommended values are changed to make "old" medicines recommendable to new users. A new term has been introduced, pre-hypertension, or precursor to high blood pressure. High blood pressure has been defined as 140/90 for a long time. In 2003, the diagnosis of pre-hypertension was established as a blood pressure of around 120/80 and 140/90.[14] This means, of course, that, by creating a new category of illness, pharmaceutical companies have gained many new customers. We observe the same thing with statins. This medication was previously given only to people with heart problems. Eventually, people were persuaded that this was a medicine suitable to all. In 2004, an expert panel accepted the recommendations for lowering of cholesterol levels from the National Institute of Health, through the National Cholesterol Education program.

After these new guidelines were recommended and approved, it was revealed that eight out of nine panel members had a financial connection to companies that produce statins! In 2006, a scientific review of these recommendations was conducted and published in the *Annals of Internal Medicine*. The review stated that no clinical evidence was found that supported the current recommendations of treatment goals for LDL cholesterol. The recommended practice of increasing the dosage in order to reach a desired value lacked enough scientific evidence to be either advantageous or safe.[15]

There are also studies published in prestigious journals that point out the absence of any positive effects of statins, despite their numerous side effects. In 2007, a study was presented in *The Lancet*—a prestigious medical journal. The study claimed that treatment based on statins was not effective in reducing the risk of death. The study also revealed that statins as a treatment only minimally reduced the risk for cardiovascular disorders. Every medication on the market has an NNT (number needed to treat) rating. This is a measurement of the number of people that must take the medication for one person to benefit. For statins, sixty-seven people have to be treated in five years with statins so one person can experience a positive result. No advantages of statin usage among women were found at all.[16] In addition to being quite ineffective, statins are a category of medicine that has a large amount of negative side effects. Why are so many on statins and why do physicians continue to prescribe them? I think you will find the answer in the $20 billion spent each year.

More weapons do not lead to less war. More jails do not lead to less crime. More money within health care (read "sick care") does not necessarily lead to better health. Which medicines or operations will solve the current health challenges? Do you believe that those who become sick have forgotten to take their medicine or remove a body part? I am shocked when I read about people who have removed their breasts and ovaries due to having genes that predispose them to cancer. We all have genes that predispose us to a range of serious diseases, but the genes can be seen as on and off switches, where we don't want to turn on the ones that can lead to disease and misery (read more about genes later in the book). What will be next? Will someone remove their arms in fear of a broken arm or simply quit trying to have a child in the fear that the child sooner or later will experience something bad?

If health care workers in the "maintenance business," like chiropractors, acupuncturists, homeopaths, osteopaths, physiotherapists, coaches, nutritionists, and training instructors, are evaluated based on our ability to extinguish fires, it is not unexpected that we don't receive a larger influence when it comes to people's health. We are not experts in extinguishing fires. We are experts in how to build and maintain a good foundation so that we can prevent fires.

If you have destroyed roof tiles or rotten wallboards in your house, wouldn't it be more natural to call a carpenter than to call the fire department?

Many will argue that the allopathic thought process is correct, since life expectancy has increased substantially in the last hundred years. Critics, on the other hand, will claim that this cannot be due to allopathic medicine but, rather, to better nutrition, sanitation, and other lifestyle factors.[17]

In order to obtain better health, we have to understand that we are programmed for good health, not disease and misery. Genes have not changed in forty thousand years. However, cardiovascular diseases, cancer, and diabetes were exceptionally rare in our ancestors. What has changed?

We have to realize that we are a living ecosystem. Unnatural things supplied to the body will never bring us closer to homeostasis. I want to bring up an example, which I overheard at a café while I worked on this book. I think this example illustrates aspects of the situation today.

A married couple and a friend, who was about sixty years old, sat at a neighboring table. The couple seemed to be in good health with normal body composition. Their friend was overweight, and when she walked, I observed that she had also difficulties walking.

The man described how he had lost ten kilograms and that his cholesterol dropped from 8 (considered high) to 4 (considered as normal) after he switched to a low-carbohydrate diet. He explained that he'd previously used statins, which had lowered his cholesterol but, in addition, had given him side effects. Now, since stopping the statins, the side effects were gone.

The friend was extremely critical and highlighted evidence in the form of evidence-based research. The man was humble enough to say that he was not sure about evidence, but he explained in an understandable and knowledgeable way the effects carbohydrates have on the body, in contrast to fat. He explained even how the environment has an effect on genetic expression and that genes were not preprogrammed for disease. He explained it brilliantly, and I almost wanted to kiss the man. The discussion lasted no more than ten minutes, but the atmosphere went noticeably bad. The couple and the friend hardly said goodbye when they left the café.

It is obvious that there are more and more people taking an active role in their own health. I think one of the primary reasons is that information is more easily accessible today than it was some years ago. The problem with the easily accessible information and exchange of opinions is that this information often comes without instructions. It can be difficult to interpret and understand without the proper context. In some cases, because of the sheer volume of information available, some people only read a headline or a small part of the latest article. Without the context, this leaves many in a defensive position. No one likes to hear he or she is wrong or has made a poor decision. Later in this book, I will properly address why it is difficult to change viewpoints and lifestyles.

Another interesting aspect of this conversation, which I will also come back to in detail, is the request for evidence. On one side of the table sits what seems to be a healthy individual with apparently normal body structure talking about a change in lifestyle that led to an improvement in his health, and on the other side sat a friend who was overweight and apparently having mobility issues, believing that her friend's change in lifestyle was not good enough evidence. This I find very interesting!

"The world as we created it is a process of our thinking. It cannot be changed without changing our thinking" (Albert Einstein).

1

Philosophy

A peek back in time: From spiritual to mechanistic

The earth has been through five mass extinctions, all caused by factors outside of humankind's control. Many believe that we are on our way to a sixth mass extinction. However, the most significant difference this time is that humankind is the creator. Bruce Lipton, a cell biologist, says, "There is bad news and there is good news. The bad news is that civilization, as we know it, is on the verge of extinction. The good news is that civilization, as we know it, is on the verge of extinction."

In order to understand why we are where we are today and why we should take action, it can be smart to take a peek back in time.

When it comes to the existential questions, archaeologists and historians have divided history into four paradigms—animism, polytheism, monotheism, and materialism. These paradigms can be defined as mutual unwritten rules.

History can be illustrated simply with a pendulum, where the outer points represent a spiritual view on one side and a mechanistic view on the other.

Animism assumedly has its roots back to 8000 BC. The pendulum points down, in between the spiritual and material, because animism is based on spirits existing in everything and emphasizes the harmony between the spiritual and material reality. Animism claims humans are children of the earth (the material) and the heavens (the spiritual). We are here to take care of and manage the Garden of Eden. We will live in harmony with nature.

Around 2000 BC, polytheism took over. This was a direction towards the spiritual. Polytheism is a belief in, or the worship of, several gods. The Greek gods characterize this epoch. Polytheism claims that humans were created out of chaos. It emphasizes the reality of blindly following the gods and living by their rules and laws.

The pendulum moves outwardly towards the spiritual side. Around 800 BC, monotheism developed. Now there is only one God, and this God controlled everything. Those who lived in compliance with God arrived in paradise, while others of another belief ended up in hell. It is in this epoch that Christianity grew considerably. The spiritual view was extremely strong.

In the 1500s, questions were raised about spiritual reality. The pendulum is heading towards the mechanistic side.

Well known names, such as Descartes, Bacon, and Newton appear a little later. The stage is set for the materialistic, reductionist, and deterministic viewpoints that, unfortunately, continue to characterize our current society.

The scientific paradigm we base our understanding on today builds on observations we can see, touch, and measure. Three aspects from Newton's philosophy from the 1700s are emphasized:

- Materialism – The universe can be understood from its visible parts.
- Reductionism – Regardless of how complex something is, an element can be pulled apart and studied in isolation.
- Determinism – The universe can be explained using a linear approach, where A leads to B, which leads to C, and so on. Exactly as in a mechanical clockwork, we can see that gear A leads to gear B occurring in a defined direction, which again leads to gear C rotating in its own direction.

We will now see how these principles have been applied to define today's "scientific truths."

Darwin was wrong

The finding of fossils implies that single-celled organisms such as bacteria, algae, and amoeba were the first forms of life on our planet.

Around 750 million years ago, these single-celled organisms began to join to form multiple-celled organisms. Initially, these single-celled organisms came together with other single-celled organisms and created their own colonies. All these single-celled organisms had the same function. This can be seen as an evolutionary trait in order to increase the chance of survival.

When cells bind themselves together, they increase their attention to their surroundings, something that is essential in order to survive. Another advantage of coming together was to save energy. For example, it takes less energy per person to move a heavy object from point A to point B when there are more people to do it.

Eventually, there were so many cells that it was no longer favorable that all had the same purpose. This led to a new evolutionary trait. In order to survive, multiple-celled organisms developed cell structure. Different cells developed special characteristics. For example, some cells specialized in sending and receiving information (nerve cells), some specialized in defending (immune cells), while others specialized in movement (muscle cells), and so on. By developing different characteristics, organisms have an even bigger chance of survival, and it requires even less energy.

We find ourselves with the same pattern in our society, with specialized tasks that combine in cooperation. We have farmers and anglers who provide our food. We have garbage men who get rid of our waste. We have police to keep peace and order. We have health personnel who take care of our health, and so on and so forth. It would have been unfavorable if everyone had the same purpose in society.

This is, however, not in line with Darwin's theory of "survival of the fittest." If the principle of survival of the fittest were the case, before cells began to join over 700 million years ago, the single-celled organisms would have fought against each other with the result that only the strongest survived. However, not even animals follow the principal of survival of the fittest. A lion does not go after a trophy animal when it hunts. The lion picks out the weakest animal that gives the least amount of resistance and biggest energy yield as possible. The sick and the injured will typically be on top of the list. To kill the sick animals will prevent them from bringing their diseases to the next generation. It is an important part of maintaining a healthy population. It is exactly in this way Wallace built his evolutionary theory at the same time as Darwin. He believed that evolution was driven by the elimination of the weakest. There is a significant difference between the elimination of the weakest and survival of the fittest.

Darwin also believed that traits were inherited from generation to generation. This led to a quest for the genetic hereditary material. In 1910, we managed, through microscopic analysis, to identify that hereditary material was found in the chromosomes in the cell nucleus.

In 1944, researchers further discovered that this hereditary material was found in DNA.[18] In this attempt, DNA was taken out from bacteria A and put in bacteria B. This showed that bacteria B received characteristics of bacteria A. The conclusion was that DNA controlled the outcome. The foundation of genetic determinism was established.

The genome theory: A dead hypothesis that is still very much alive

Watson and Crick continued to work with genetic determinism. They found that the DNA molecule consists of different nitrogen bases (adenine, thymine, cytosine, and guanine). The sequences of the nitrogen bases control the sequences of which amino acids are created and, with that, which proteins are formed. These long chains of DNA can be separated in individual genes, which function as blueprints to different proteins.

Watson and Crick also explained how DNA consists of two chains that encircle one another, where one is a copy of the other (double helix). They believed that, when these chains split up, they copied themselves. This copy is called RNA. Their gene hypothesis was that DNA controlled RNA that controls which proteins will be created. The proteins control the different characteristics. Since we cannot choose our genes, we are, then, victims of our heritage.

Since the discovery of the genetic code by Crick and Watson in 1953, there has been a belief that the DNA inherited from our parents has determined our traits and characteristics. This conventional view on genes also make us believe that our inherited program is fixed, without the opportunity to change or influence it. It makes us believe that genes function as a "read-only" computer program. We can today prove that this is not true. Through epigenetic research, we have proved that the same blueprint of DNA can create as much as thirty thousand different variations of proteins, which again is controlled by the surroundings.[19]

Epigenetics is a new direction that has emerged. *Epi* means "above," and epigenetics means "above the genes," or in other words, what controls the genes. This new knowledge radically changes how we see what controls our lives.[20] Genes do not control our fate. Your genes can certainly predispose you to various conditions like ADHD, cancer, obesity, or substance abuse, but a piano can certainly predispose you to play wrong notes as well. Genes are good, but there is always a chance of a mutation that turns the gene bad. The blueprint from the genetic material, which is inherited and goes from family member to family member, is impressionable and can be changed. Genes can be "expressed," or in other words, can be toggled on and off based on the signals from the environment around us— an environment consisting of, perhaps, stress, chemicals, unhealthy food, poisons, viruses, and so on. Other times, these signals come from within the body (outside of the cell), for example by different states of mind (anger, happiness, relief, frustration, and so on).

It is not always possible to control what happens in the environment on the outside of the body, but your choice of how to react to the environment on the outside influences how you are on the inside. The environment of your cells influences your genes. Since you can influence how you perceive the environment from outside of the body, you can influence the inner states and environment around the cell inside the body. Ultimately, it means that you determine your genetic fate!

You were born to use your genes, not the other way around.

Newer research shows the environment influences 90 percent of the genes (K. Richardson). "In reality, genes contribute to our characteristics but do not determine them."[21]

The new understanding of what regulates our biology can be portrayed as such: Our senses interpret the environment and send signals to the DNA. Our DNA will use that information to determine what type of RNA needs to be made and, thus, which proteins need to be made. These proteins give us our characteristics and character traits.

Let us look a little bit closer at this phenomenon, without going too much into detail. In 1960, gene researcher Howard Temin published his studies, which recommend that RNA can influence the cell's DNA. It was unpopular to go against the gene hypothesis that had come to be embraced so warmly, despite that it never had been something other than a hypothesis. It's ironic when a definition in conventional medicine is applied science!

Despite a lot of fuss around Temin's findings, he received the Nobel Peace Prize in physiology in 1975 for discovering reversible transcriptase enzymes that copy RNA information inside the DNA code. The environment around the cell influences DNA that signals which kind of proteins will be made, which in turn controls our different characteristics.

We can see this with polar bears, for example. From the "old" gene hypothesis model, which many continue to support, the belief is that it was the individuals who were best equipped to survive in the Arctic regions who passed on their genes to the next generation. The fittest polar bears, according to the gene hypothesis, had genes that coded for specific proteins that created thicker fur. Obviously, the polar bears that did not have thick fur would die, without the possibility of passing on their genes. There is much to suggest that this explanation is wrong. Recent research points to the environment, specifically the cold climate, as sending signals to the cells, which again sends signals to the genes to produce proteins in order to make thick fur.

For humanity, this is exceptional. It means that we can influence our genes to produce the proteins that are purposeful for the situation or environment we find ourselves in. We are not victims of our heritage after all! The bad news is that we can no longer blame our parents that we are not satisfied with the way we are.

A study from Sweden published in 2013 shows that seven thousand genes had changed character after a six-month period where twenty-three slightly overweight men, trained spinning and doing aerobics twice a week on average. This constitutes almost 30 percent of all the genes we have.[22]

In other words, genes are changeable!

In 1990, the Human Genome Project was launched on behalf of the US National Institute of Health. The goal was to identify all of the genes to all human characteristics and traits. When this was done, the pharmaceutical industry would be able to create medicines that could match the "defective" genes that gave undesired traits. With over 100,000 proteins in the human body, the researchers expected to find at least 100,000 different genes. To their amazement and frustration, they managed to uncover only around 25,000 genes.[23] In comparison, the nematode *Caenorhabditis elegans* (a primitive worm) consists of around 969 cells and around 24,000 genes (against 50 trillion human cells).[24]

A banana fly, which is considerably more complex than a nematode contains around 15,000 genes.[25] Mice, which are often used in research, have around the same amount of genes as humans.

How can it be that humans have only 1,000 to 1,500 more genes than a primitive nematode?

For the pharmaceutical industry, the fall of the genome theory is extremely bad news.

Despite that the gigantic Human Genome Project appeared to be completely wrong, a huge portion of the population still believes in genetic determinism. Every day, health providers who believe in genetic determinism tell you that, with medicine, you can rid yourselves of your bothers and, best of all, you can continue to live like before! Isn't that what happens when you are recommended medication for high blood pressure, cholesterol medicine, painkillers, anti-inflammatory medicine, or more commonly diets! We are being led to believe that it is not our fault. It is the genes that have led us into misery, and there is nothing we can do about it, other than take medicine and continue to live like before.

In an article published by the Norwegian Institute of Public Health in 2012, we can read, "The use of blood pressure medication in Norway has increased by almost 5 times in 30 years.[26]

Furthermore, "The increase in the usage of blood pressure medication is probably due to the combination of better diagnostic of high blood pressure, lower boundaries for startup of treatment and more intense treatment, says the senior advisor at the Norwegian Institute of Public Health."

It is a known strategy of the pharmaceutical industry to change the recommended values in order to sell more of the same medicine. An example of this is pre-hypertension, which I have mentioned earlier.

Furthermore, "It is important to follow the recommendation of prescribed drugs in society. In that way, we can get a hold of trends before they develop in an unfortunate direction. The increase in the use of blood pressure medicine can indicate that the population now is being treated better," says the same senior advisor at the Norwegian Institute of Public Health.

It is emphasized that a good compliance of blood pressure treatment is important in order to reduce the risk of heart attacks and stroke.

Neither the article itself nor the studies it refers to say anything about the cause of hypertension. It underlines, rather, the reality of having to continue with medication forever, without changing anything else! Such statements substantiate my stance that genetic determinism continues to stand strongly in our public health care system. I wonder, Is it so that Norwegian Institute of Public Health (public health care) believes that the lack of blood pressure medicine in the body is a cause of higher blood pressure levels or due to a genetic failure?

A woman in her fifties consulted me because she had pain behind her left shoulder blade.

Before she visited me, she consulted her doctor; she was anxious it could be a heart attack. Her doctor sent her to hospital. The only thing that was found during the examination was that her blood pressure was a little high, something I would have attributed as normal when you are checked in at the hospital for a possible heart attack. When she was under observation, a nurse came in during her visiting round in order to give medicine. The nurse was surprised that the woman did not take any medicine and offered her soothing medication or at least something to make her sleep. The woman kindly rejected the offer. After a short while, the doctor came and asked the woman to take cholesterol medicine and blood pressure medicine. After all, she had checked into the hospital under suspicion of having a heart attack.

Despite unsubstantial findings, she was sent home with cholesterol and blood pressure medicine in her purse, without any other information other than that everything seemed okay. She suffered, after a short period, a range of side effects. She consulted her doctor, who took her off the cholesterol medicine. She became better very quickly.

During a consultation with me, I asked her more specifically about her blood pressure. A twenty-four-hour measurement of her blood pressure was never conducted. When she was tested at the hospital and by her doctor, the overpressure was right up to 140 (which borders on hypertension). She also informed me that, based on previous measurements taken at home, her blood pressure could fluctuate from under normal levels to levels for hypertension—not unlike how blood pressure works, if you ask me.

Think back to your basic philosophy, which I talked about initially. If we agree that life brings health on nature's premises, then the Norwegian Institute of Public Health's recommendations are contradictory to the basic philosophy and will be destructive. If, on the other hand, you believe that we are created for disease and misery, the reasoning from the National Institute of Public Health will be correct, and the recommendations will be recommendable.

You have to make up your own mind about what you think is correct.

I participated in a seminar in 2012 in the United States of America. I remember especially well during the stay that a commercial constantly popped up on TV and various billboards. It was about a revolutionary pill that could guarantee you would lose weight without a need to change your lifestyle. I remember thinking, *We cannot be that stupid!* When I tell people about this advertisement, most of the reactions are the same.

Furthermore, I would like to ask, Is there really such a big difference between this type of diet pill and a blood pressure-reducing or cholesterol-reducing pill?

Stem cells: They do what they are told to do

A stem cell is a cell with the original genetic material. Stem cells are undifferentiated biological cells with raw potential. When the cells are activated, they will develop into what the body has a need for, such as muscle cells, nerve cells, bone cells, immune cells, or skin cells. While inside a fetus in the mother's womb, they are embryo cells. When one is born, they are called stem cells.

In stem cell research, a cell with the original genetic material is cloned. A stem cell is cultivated in a petri dish and separates itself around every ten hours. Within one week, there are fifty thousand stem cells that are identical to the parent cell.

Bruce Lipton, a cell biologist, already conducted studies on stem cells in 1967. These studies are simple but describe important mechanisms.

A description of his experiment—when a group of stem cells are placed in a certain medium in a petri dish, these cells can develop into muscle cells, for example. If another group of stem cells from the same group as the first example are placed in another type of medium in a petri dish, they can develop into nerve cells. When a third group of stem cells are placed in a third medium in a petri dish, these cells can develop into bone cells.

The exact same cells develop into different cells in different mediums. This means that it is not genes that determine the outcome, but the environment! This simple experiment proves again that genetic determinism is wrong.

Furthermore, research shows that, if a healthy cell is placed in a sick environment, then the healthy cell will become sick. It will protect itself, stop growing and developing, and then eventually die. If a sick cell is placed in a healthy environment, the sick cell can become better again. It will begin to repair itself and eventually grow and develop.

Humans are comprised of around 50 trillion cells. We can look at this as a big petri dish surrounded by skin. The blood is the medium in this big petri dish, and the brain decides what the blood will contain. Through sensations (perception), the brain will interpret the incoming signals and produce its own response to make the biochemistry in our blood. This decides the fate of the cells.

For example, if you receive a groin strain, this will start a response that changes your inner chemical composition and, furthermore, sends signals to the genes from the outside of the cells. The genes interpret this signal and create proteins, which are in accordance with the signal.

These proteins give a message to the stem cells about changing to healthier muscle cells so that the muscle can heal. The stem cells just waits for a signal for what it will be used for. In this instance, it was the local trauma that overloaded the muscle. Millions of such processes occur in your body continuously.

Again, back to basic philosophy—if you believe that the body's auto regulation is wrong, which leads toward disease and misery, medicine and surgery would be your solution. The contrary view is that medicines and surgery would be contradictory and destructive if you don't need sick care.

Every day, we lose hundreds of thousands of cells. These are replaced by the information from the stem cells. For example, if we have destroyed cells in the pancreas, an optimally functioning body will replace these with new well-functioning cells. If this does not happen, conventional medicine might regard it as a dysfunction of the stem cells, and the goal will be to replace old stem cells with new ones. This type of mechanistic and reductionist view does not take into consideration the environment or energies; nor does it consider the brain's function. What will happen to these new stem cells if they receive the same signals as the old ones, which led to dysfunction of the pancreas?

What if we develop a disease that is lifestyle related? Our lifestyle sends bad signals to the stem cells. Would it help to supply the body with new stem cells? There is usually nothing wrong with the stem cells. The problem is not the stem cells; it's the signals from an unhealthy environment.

Evolution is not random

In a letter written by Darwin to Moritz Wagner in 1876, Darwin wrote, "In my opinion, the greatest error which I have committed has been not allowing sufficient weight to the direct action of the surroundings, i.e. food, climate, etc., independently of natural selection."

By mutations and epigenetic modifications, primitive cells have managed to choose and change their own genetic code, so they become more adaptable to their environment. In contrast to Darwin's theory that evolution is random, new science believes that evolution represents a meaningful process. Individuals survive by adapting to the environment and are driven by becoming a part of a society.

A study published in 1999 stated that evolution is not random. Rather, it is a direct influence of the surroundings. The way the researchers showed this was by studying microbes over time. They placed microbes in different test tubes and followed the evolution of the bacteria in every tube through 24,000 generations. Researchers found that these miniature changes happened in the exact same way completely down to ATCG (nitrogen bases) sequences in DNA, caused by the same environmental signals.[27]

The germ theory: Good for the pharmaceutical industry, bad for humans

During the last four centuries, conventional medicine has had a lasting belief in Newton's philosophy, stating that matter controls its own fate. Ever since Descartes's period in the 1700s, the cause of disease in matter has been pursued.

Around the same time Darwin postulated his evolutionary theory, the English physicist John Snow discovered that cholera was caused by something in the drinking water.[28] Shortly after, the French microbiologist Louis Pasteur also claimed an existing connection between disease and microorganisms.[29]

Forty years after John Snow's findings, Robert Koch developed his postulations that disease was created from particular microorganisms.[30]

In addition to the bacteria theory fitting in well with the materialistic viewpoint, it also fits in very well with Darwin's survival of the fittest. It is either the bacteria or you. We are constantly told that deadly bacteria and viruses are next in line. Recent examples of this are bird flu, swine flu, Ebola, and the Zika virus.

The French physiologist Claude Bernard disagreed with Pasteur's theory of bacteria. "Illnesses hover constantly above us, their seeds blown by the wind, but they do not set in the terrain unless the terrain is ready to receive them," articulated Bernard. While Pasteur meant "the seed" in itself was the cause of disease, Bernard meant it was the earth in which the seed eventually would grow up that was the problem.

There is no doubt that bacteria can inflict serious diseases and, in worse cases, death. Some of you who read this book would maybe not have been here today if it was not for conventional medicine fighting these bacteria. Still, it is important to emphasize that the cause is not in the bacteria itself. If these bacteria did not have favoring surroundings to grow up in, they would never exist. It is not foolish to dry the floor after a leak from the roof, but it would be foolish not to repair the roof.

"While giving lip service to the importance of preventive health care, the medical profession put most of its eggs in the germ-theory basket. Microbes were the great cause of disease. Nutritious diet, adequate rest, clean air and water, regular exercise, proper posture and the alleviation of stressful living were of little clinical import. The patient became passive as the doctor became active. The patient was the innocent victim of a 'bug'; it was up to the physician to find it and kill it".[31]

Ninety percent of the body's cells are microbes. Most of the microbes are essential for us to survive. While modern medicine, based on the germ theory, has focused on the war against bacteria for more than a century, we are now learning how to live in harmony with them.

"If the germ theory of disease were correct there would be no one living to believe it."[32]

Newton versus Einstein

In 1895, an equivalent theory came to the materialistic, reductionist, and deterministic thought process. Conrad Roentgen discovered the x-ray. This proved the existence of an invisible force made from matter, which could penetrate another matter. Simultaneously, Antoine Becquerel, and then later on Marie and Pierre Curie, discovered something called radioactivity. Shortly after, the British physicist Sir Joseph John Thomson discovered the electron that disproved that the atom was the smallest unit as Newton claimed (reductionism).

The German physicist Max Planck discovered that electrons could jump from one shell to another, where they travel from one energy level to another. This was the start of quantum physics. In 1905, the German physicist Albert Einstein could show that nonmaterial light could express physical characteristics. Einstein developed his well-known formula E=mc2, which shows that atoms are not made of matter but of energy!

Science today tells us that an atom contains a large amount of subatomic particles such as quarks, bosons (photons), and fermions (electrons and protons). Quantum physics depicts an atom as a minitornado. Materials or humans, for that matter, are comprised of X amount of minitornados. Think about a tornado the way we see it as a weather phenomenon; if it had not been for all the debris, it would be invisible. If we had driven straight into an invisible tornado without matter, it would still feel like driving into a brick wall.

"The field is the sole governing agency of the particle," Einstein claimed. We must look at the energy field as what controls matter. A simple example I remember from high school is when we sprinkle iron particles over a piece of paper with and without a magnet underneath. Without the magnet, we will observe that the iron particles fall into a random pattern, while with a magnet under the paper, a very specific and defined pattern is created.

Let's look at another example. You have probably been sunburned. How could this have been possible if it had not been for the energy from the sun?

Energy in one form or another is the common denominator for everything in our lives. If we try to understand the reality without taking into consideration the invisible energy that exists, we will fail.

When we look at atoms as energy, we are talking about wavelengths and volts, not mass and weight, as it is in Newtown's principles. Einstein's conclusion E=mc2 proves that energy and matter are one and the same.

Humans consist of trillions of cells that contain molecules. The molecules contain the atoms. These atoms consist of electrons, protons, and neutrons, which are energy. Light reflects when it meets energy. What we see through our eyes in reality is actually illusion of light.

Hundreds of studies in the last ten years have shown that invisible energies control our biology. Specific frequencies and electromagnetic radiation regulates DNA, RNA, protein synthesis, cell division, endocrine functions, nerve functions, and so on.[33]

The speed of electromagnetic energy is 300,000 km per second, whereas the speed of signals of hormones, neurotransmitters, or growth factor is less than 1 cm per second.[34]

The fact that the body is a mechanism that demands faster reaction should be an indication that medicine, with its slower chemoreceptors, cannot possibly be the most optimal solution toward good health.

Magnetoencephalography (MEG) can read the brain's energy patterns a good distance away from the body. This proves that the brain's activity is sent out to the surroundings in the same way that sound waves are sent from a tuning fork.

A study published in 2006 shows how the brain can register an incoming event. Test subjects were hooked up to electronic devices that register emotional reactions. They were shown a series of pictures, most of them peaceful and harmonic, except for around 3 percent, which contained shocking violence or sex. What was interesting was that the test subjects registered an emotional response seconds before the shocking pictures were shown on the screen.

Another study created by a doctor, Larry Dossey, evaluated sixty scientific studies that could prove that prayer had a significant effect on healing and recovery.[35] He also discovered that prayer had little effect or no effect, if one did not have any passion behind the prayer.

I recognize this from my clinical experience every day. In order to be helping others, it is essential to truly desire the best for the patient. If you as a health practitioner are not doing well yourself, or maybe you feel even worse than the patient you are helping, I think it is difficult to achieve good results. When you help someone, you must have something to give. The energy flow must go in the right direction.

2

Body and Mind

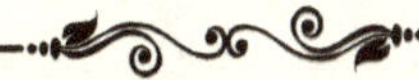

The Cell

The structure of a cell

We find our genes in the cell nucleus. As a counterbalance to genetic determinism, where genes control our destiny, researchers have found that cells can survive for more than two months without a nucleus and without DNA (enucleation).[36]

These sensational findings have previously been ignored. The first attempts to demonstrate removing the nucleus and genetic material from the cell were already conducted over hundred years ago. It is admittedly not free from problems for a cell to live without genes; the cell will no longer be able to divide itself, reproduce, or replace proteins that naturally die.

If the nucleus does not function as the cell's brain, what is it then? Interestingly, studies show that a cell cannot survive without the cell membrane.

Prokaryotic cells represent life in its most primitive form. Such cells, which include bacteria and other microbes, contain only a cell membrane and a little cytoplasm inside of the cell. The cell membrane is only 1/7 millionth of a millimeter thick. We were not able to observe the cell membrane until the electron microscope was developed after World War II. Although a prokaryotic cell is extremely simple, it shows its intelligence.

It does not have, like more advanced eukaryotic cells, organelles such as a nucleus or mitochondria. We know that the prokaryotic cell eats, digests, grows, forms, protects itself, gets rid of impurities, and so on. It seems as though the cell membrane plays an important role.

A membrane has three thin layers. The inner and outer layers contain phospholipids. These phospholipids consist of both polar and nonpolar molecules. Polar molecules have either a negative or a positive charge and will thus attract/repel other molecules with the same charge. Polar molecules are water soluble, while nonpolar molecules are comprised of fat and can't dissolve in water. The phosphate part of phospholipid is polar and water-soluble, while the lipid part is nonpolar and does not dissolve in water. The lipid part inside the membrane will not allow molecules with positive or negative charges through it. This is an effective isolator for preventing all molecules to penetrate inside the cell. Since the lipids prevent molecules from penetrating the cell, the cell needs other mechanisms in order to allow important information to slip through.

Receptors are what make the membrane so special and important, as they are proteins with different charges that attract or repel other molecules. There exist many different receptors, but they can roughly be separated as receptor proteins and effector proteins.

Receptor proteins are the cell's sensory apparatus. They can either sit on the outside and react to specific signals from the outside or sit on the inside and react to the conditions within the cell. Studies show that receptor proteins do not react just to physical signals, but also to energies such as sound, light, and other invisible signals.[37]

Effector proteins have other specific tasks. For example, they can be transporter proteins, which ensure that molecules are transported from the outside to the inside of the cell membrane. They can be enzymes, which have the task of breaking down molecules. They can be proteins, which take care of the cell's movement and form.

If this was a bit difficult to understand, let us compare the cell membrane to a football stadium. The stadium or fence acts as phospholipids, preventing people from coming in. The guards at the ticket check function as receptor proteins. If you can show a ticket, you will be allowed inside. If you do not have a ticket or you have a fake ticket, you will be denied entry. Similarly a molecule passes receptors proteins and is allowed into the cell in order to perform its purposeful task. In the cell, football players illustrate the genes. The outcome of the game is not determined, in opposition to the way deterministic conventional medicine looks at genes. Every player and every team has numerous opportunities in order to achieve a result (this is also so with genes). Their performance is influenced by information from the outside, for example the weather, the coach, the spectators, the atmosphere, and on and on. It is also influenced by what happens on the pitch (equivalent to what happens inside the cell)—which team scores the first goal, injuries, interactions, and so on.

A cell's life is specific to the characteristic of adjusting itself to a dynamic environment. Since the genes cannot preprogram a cell's life, this means that the cell membrane, in reality, determines the fate of the cell and, in effect, is the cell's brain.

Supporting research is the same as that conducted with the nucleus (enucleation), except that, in this case, the cell membrane is removed. Because the cell is completely dependent on the signals from the environment, a cell will immediately become "brain dead" or comatose as soon as the cell membrane, receptor proteins, or effector proteins are removed.

From an evolutionary perspective, we have talked about prokaryotic, single-celled organisms developing into eukaryotic, multiple-celled organisms with specific tasks and groupings (organelles). This has been a developmental trait to increase the attention to the surroundings, save energy, improve the defense mechanism, and increase the chance of survival. This developmental trait can be seen in context with the cell membrane. Since the cell membrane is the cell's "brain," an increase in the cell membrane's area will lead to an increased attention to the surroundings. When parts of the cell membrane went into the cell and created intracellular organelles, enclosed with its own cell membrane, this increased the cell membrane's area substantially.

For those of you who have a technical background rather than a biological background, it can help if I describe a cell's function with a computer analogy. (Keep in mind, this analogy is mechanical and is much simplified compared to the human body.) To put it simply, a computer is built of hardware—the physical components of a computer. Hardware cannot function alone, and it depends on software or an operating system in order for us to do something beneficial on the computer. We also need a keyboard to type different commands. If we look at this as an analogy with humans, the signals from the environment will be that which give the commands to the keyboard. The receptors in the cell membrane are like the computer's keyboard. Effector proteins are like the computer's CPU (central processing unit). DNA is like a hard disk. When signals go from the effector proteins to the DNA, the genes inside of the DNA's double helix will decide which proteins need to be made.

We can regard the cell's nucleus, including genetic material, as an external hard drive. We can also see the similarities between cells being able to survive without the nucleus as a computer with its external hard drive being removed as long as information is downloaded onto the active memory.

Most computers come with the same software when we buy it, in the same way humans are conceived with the same possibilities/characteristics. As time goes by, different people will download different programs. The hard disk remains the same, but dependent on what type of program is downloaded, the computer will perform very different tasks with different results.

Most importantly in this comparison is that both humans and computers are programmable. Our genes do not predetermine our fate, just as the computer is not predetermined by its hardware, but by which commands it is given. In relation to computers, they are dependent on the commands from humans. In relation to humans or the simple cells, we are dependent on the environment.

A Spanish study, presented in the proceedings of the National Academy of Science, USA, in 2005, demonstrated the importance of the environment.[38]

The study shows that forty pairs of identical twins (born with the same genotype) from the ages of three to seventy-four developed differently, especially as time went by. Younger twins with similar lifestyles who had lived several years together had relatively similar genetic expression, while older twins with more different lifestyles and who did not live together had a very different genetic expression. The study showed that a fifty-year-old pair of twins had four times as many different gene expressions as a three-year-old pair of twins. Several studies have also shown that adopted children received the same type of cancer as their adoptive parents.

A very important difference between the brain and the computer is that the computer does not have emotions to interpret the commands. The computer does not understand context. If you are sad or depressed and hear a "happy" song on the radio, you might turn it off. If you are happy, you might turn up the volume instead. It is the same song, but you act differently. Food will most likely taste better if you are hungry, compared to when you are feeling full. If you like to enjoy a glass of wine, you have probably noticed that you will have different experiences with the same type of wine in different settings.

When you type in a command on the keyboard, the computer will do exactly what you tell it to do. If you have typed only one letter wrong, the computer will not understand.

Growth or protection

Millions of cells die every day in your body. In order to survive, a cell must ensure both growth and protection. Studies show that a cell cannot provide growth and development simultaneously while it protects itself.[39] When nutrients are placed in front of a cell, it will open up and move toward the nutrients. When a poisonous medium is placed in front of a cell, the cell will close itself off and move away from the threatening environment.

In a human body consisting of 50 trillion cells, it is not so that all of the cells will be involved in either growth or protection, such as in single-celled organisms. You can survive stressful situations, but stress over time will lead to impaired vitality.

To develop ourselves, it is not enough to avoid situations that put us in defense mode. We must actively seek situations that stimulate growth and development. If you travel by car, plane, or another form of transportation, you have probably noticed that you become tired after a while. If rest solely led to more energy, why do you become tired, just by sitting?

You are created for movement, not inactivity. In the same way, your brain is created to be stimulated. You have probably also noticed that you become mentally tired by doing nothing. Statistics on sick leave clearly show that the longer an employee is away from work, the less chance he or she has to return. The body and the brain become more and more tired if they are not stimulated.

Your body and brain are able to prioritize. An everyday example can be observed when the fire alarm goes off when you are eating.

When you eat, this is a process that goes in the direction of growth and maintenance. If you suddenly hear a fire alarm, your body will automatically inhibit digestion, growth, and maintenance. The only thing that matters now is protection. It does not matter whether you can break down food in a good way if you get caught in a fire and die. The body redirects the signals to the skeletal muscles and the heart, so that you can run away as fast as possible.

Ideally, we are created in order to use our energy to grow and reproduce in the most energy efficient way possible. Our defense system is only made for being used over a short period of time and demands a lot of energy. Much of the energy we use for growth and development will give us a positive net energy balance, while energy used to protect ourselves would not give anything back. When we also know that the body prioritizes protection over growth and development, we can think about what happens to the body when many nowadays live under constant stress and protection twenty-four hours a day, seven days a week.

Fear, pessimism, competition, anger, frustration, hostility, or concern will not send signals to the genes regarding better health. On the contrary, these inputs turn up the defense system and make the body ready for a full state of readiness. There are studies, which show that signals, which tells the stem cells what to do, become highly disturbed under stress. The body does not heal properly and worst-case can lead to unfortunate and improper responses such as uncontrolled cell division (cancer).

The Nervous System

The body's defense system

We can divide our defense system into two different systems.

One system protects us against external threats. This is called HPA axis, which stands for hypothalamic–pituitary–adrenal axis.

When the body is exposed to an external danger, we are primarily dependent on the brain to interpret this as a threat. When this happens, the hypothalamus releases corticotrophin-releasing factor (CRF) and is transported to the pituitary gland. Here, the adrenocorticotropic hormones (ACTH) are produced and transported through the blood to the adrenal glands. The adrenal glands release stress hormones, which are transported in the bloodstream (adrenaline). This leads to a range of processes to protect the body.

The blood flow is directed out into the arms and legs so that we are able to be mobile and to escape. The blood flow to the organs is reduced because growth and maintenance is no longer prioritized. Our heart rate increases, our breathing rate increases, and our blood pressure rises so that we get more nutrients out to the cells. Essential fatty acids are released, and insulin receptors are deregulated so that you can have more glucose available in the blood, which you can use for energy. The production of platelets and sticky factors increases so you will be better suited to respond to injury. Simultaneously, the intake of LDL in the liver is deregulated, along with the production of HDL. This leads to more LDL (the "bad" cholesterol) in the body and less HDL (the "good" cholesterol).

Glycogen is broken down in the liver in order to increase blood sugar. Proteins are broken down for additional energy demands. The body stores fat, and you will gain weight. You get "cravings" for fat and sugar, which, by ingestion, will increase the blood sugar, which leads to more energy.

The pancreas produces more insulin, which again produces a stress response and continues the vicious circle. The brain increases attention to sensory information. This is at the cost of memory and concentration. Examples are fibromyalgia and chronic fatigue syndrome where one becomes very sensitive to touch because he or she is under chronic stress.

This part of the defense system is effective and works quickly, but it is not made to be active over long periods of time. This system can be compared with the command "set" in "ready, set, go" before a race. When "ready" is announced, athletes loosen up, take a deep breath, and go to the starting blocks. At "set," the athletes are down in the starting blocks, and the body is waiting nervously. Adrenaline flows throughout the entire body. Just think if "go" was not announced and the athletes were left standing in a "set position."

The body would quickly become exhausted. There would definitely not be room for growth and maintenance.

In today's society, many people unfortunately live in "set mode." Our energy deteriorates by both under and overstimulation. We live linear lives, and we will not manage to recover.

Today, you are looked upon as weak if you need time to recover. There are high standards for effectiveness and perfectionism. Something must happen all the time. Take a look at waiting people at a bus stop. Do you see anyone who is not on his or her phone? There are studies that show that almost all serious diseases, which are inherited through life, are linked to chronic stress.[40]

Stress can start more than 1,400 chemical reactions and produces more than thirty hormones and neurotransmitters.[41]

In a crisis, survival is dependent on how fast your body reacts. There is a deeper function in the brain, which is one of the first areas to develop in the womb—called the amygdala, a part of the "unconscious brain." The reflective activity in the unconscious part of the brain is much faster than in the conscious part of the brain that relates to sense and logical thinking. In threatening situations, stress hormones will reduce the blood circulation to the conscious part of the brain and, therefore, its function. Hormones will increase the blood circulation to the unconscious part of the brain and make it possible with an effective fight-or-flight system. This will simultaneously make you less intelligent, since the activity in the conscious part of the brain is deprioritized.[42]

An example of this from everyday life is exam stress. When you become very nervous, your stress hormones kick in, lowering the desired activity in the frontal lobe of the brain (the conscious part of the brain). The effect is that you will be less intelligent. You will not understand the first question, become frustrated, and release even more stress hormones. You move on to the next question, which is an easy question and normally should be a walk in the park, but you can't manage to answer it because your body is in stress mode.

I was not aware of this principle until after I had finished my studies. I had to learn it the hard way. During my years at the university, I experienced that I performed much better when I was satisfied with the effort I had put down before the tests/exams. If I knew I should have done more, my performance went down. I also realized that, when I was satisfied with my effort before the exam, my attitude changed. I felt more confident and my focus was now to show off my skills. If I felt I should have prepared myself better, my focus changed to thinking about my weaker areas, and I felt the exam was there to pin me down and reveal my weaknesses.

Today I know why I suddenly performed better during exams. It was not because I had studied harder; it was more like I'd invented my basic premises for a happy life. I became more confident and was able to use my conscious mind in situations when I needed it. I have certainly taken advantage of this principle in lots of situations later in life as well.

Many studies point toward stress hormones as inhibiting the growth of nerve cells. In turn, this can lead to depression. In a 2003 study, Holden shows that the hippocampus and prefrontal cortex are actually less developed in patients under chronic stress.

We've all known that stress can influence the health in a negative way, but in 2012, a study was published showing that we possibly must rethink our perception of stress.[43]

Stress, however, can also do you some good. This study shows that your perception of stress will decide which processes your body will activate and, thus, decide whether stress is fortunate or adverse for you. This simply means that you can live an extremely hectic life, without unfavorable consequences, as long as you enjoy it.

Actually, the study shows that those who have a high level of stress but enjoy it have lower mortality rates than those with a relatively low stress level. Stress, in general, will not kill you, but you might be in trouble if you perceive stress as dangerous!

Another study published in 2012, shows that, if you think the physiological responses of stress are advantageous, you will also develop a favorable physiological response.[44]

For example, a heart that beats faster delivers more oxygen-rich blood to your muscles, a more frequent breathing rate leads to more oxygen to your brain, tunnel vision will make it easier to focus on your goal, and anxiety will make you more careful so that you do not take any chances.

A common reaction to stress is when the heart beats faster and the coronary vessels contract. This is an adverse reaction and can lead to cardiovascular disease. The interesting aspect of this study was that the test subjects who were informed that stress response made them more fit to handle stress did not experience constriction of their heart vessels. Actually, their responses strongly resembled how the heart behaved when they were happy or showed courage. When you choose to see the stress response as fortunate, you create a body composition that resembles the one for bravery. In other words, the way you experience stress can be the difference between you becoming fifty years old or ninety years old!

Another significantly interesting finding shows that stress leads to the production of the hormone oxytocin. We know this hormone as a favorable hormone. It is produced when we are social and hug someone we care very much about. The hormone is called, not without reason, "the hug hormone." When the body produces oxytocin when you are stressed, this makes you more social. You will consult others for support, love, and care.

This is not unlike single cells that come together with others in order to improve their survival characteristics in relation to evolution. In addition, oxytocin appears to be anti-inflammatory and especially helps the regeneration of heart cells so that the heart becomes stronger. Isn't it amazing that the body produces a hormone that protects us against the damaging effects stress can have in stressful situations? This hormone, in addition to what I have written about earlier, supports that we are created for wellness, not disease and misery.

Isn't it also fantastic that, in difficult situations, a hormone is produced that makes us consult others, so that we do not have to be alone with our problems? When we have such a fantastic body, is it really so wise to overrule these mechanisms with medication?

Again, we see the example that "the field is the sole governing agency of the particle." The "field" represents the mind, whereas the "particle" represents the body. The surroundings itself do not control the outcome, but the way in which you interpret your surroundings do.

PTSD (post-traumatic stress disorder) has been a well-known diagnosis for years. It impacts those who have had traumatic experiences in life. A new diagnosis has appeared in the last few years, called PTG (post-traumatic growth). It is common to hear about people saying that they have become stronger from a traumatic experience. One example is a divorce that, in the beginning, can feel very traumatic but, after a while, will make one stronger. Another example is a person overcoming a battle with a life-threatening disease. People who have survived such illnesses often say that they have gotten a different perspective on life, they have taken different choices, and life has become richer.

If you choose to see stress as a challenge, this can lead to growth and development. If you choose to see stress as a threat, the body will protect itself, and it will be harmful if the threat persists.

Our other defense system protects us against internal threats like bacteria and viruses. This is our immune system. The immune system demands its share of energy. Just think about how you felt the last time you had a cold.

The HPA system, described above, is prioritized before the immune system.

Think about having a stomach infection. The immune system will work at its fullest. If you suddenly smell smoke and hear the fire alarm, the stress hormones instantly will suppress the immune system in order to save energy. The energy is redirected so that you are able to escape the building as quickly as possible.

Stress hormones are so effective that they even are used actively in treatment with organ transplants. When an organ is transplanted, the nervous system naturally reacts by seeing the organ as a foreign body and will try to get rid of it. By administering stress hormones, medical professionals can suppress the natural tendency of the nervous system, so that the organ is not rejected.

The Mind

The conscious versus the unconscious part of the mind

Our mind has a conscious part and an unconscious part in the brain.

The conscious part is localized in the prefrontal cortex, which is an area in front of the brain and was developed more recently. This part separates us from animals or other primitive creatures. This constitutes your personality, desires, and lust. Simultaneously, it is impressionable, so that you can, to a certain degree, create your own future. The conscious part of the mind is used when you think forward or back in time. The conscious part of the mind constitutes only around 5 percent of how the mind operates.

The remaining 95 percent is the unconscious part. The unconscious part of the mind does not choose or judge. Its main function is a reflex mechanism to protect the body. An example is temperature regulation. When it becomes colder, you do not need to actively think of the body beginning to shiver or the regulation of the bloodstream to different parts of the body so that it is protected. The unconscious part of the mind works proactively and will protect us.

Another example is when the body automatically creates callus (bone substance) around a fracture so that the fracture is stabilized and can heal.

We also use the unconscious part of the mind when we do automatic activities, without having to activate the conscious part of the mind.

When you are learning to drive a car, you will, mainly, use the conscious part of the mind. You must actively think about how to use the gear and clutch and how to signal and navigate. Eventually after you have done this many times, the unconscious part of the mind gradually takes over so that the process is automatic.

If you are used to driving a car, you have probably noticed that you can drive a long distance without really noticing your surroundings. You can talk to the passenger, listen to the radio, or think about other things while simultaneously driving the car. Without the programming of the unconscious mind, this would be impossible.

How you behave when you are happy, sad, angry, nervous, or excited is mainly controlled by your unconscious mind, downloaded by observation and experience.

In the form of lectures and published findings over the course of twenty years, from 1890 to 1910, Ivan Pavlov spoke about how a stimulus leads to a learned response. Pavlov observed that dogs secreted saliva when they received food, but sometimes other factors could trigger this response as well. For example, the dog could begin to drool when hearing the footsteps of someone bringing food. Pavlov began with a systematic study of how such a signal, for example a metronome sound, could begin to trigger drooling if the metronome sound repeatedly was signaling food.

The unconscious part of the mind is programmed through the stimulus-response principle and is a million times more powerful than the conscious part of the mind.

Do you remember the example from the book about the married couple and their friend discussing nutrition? The unconscious mind, which is 95 percent of who you are, will automatically defend what you previously have downloaded through observation and experience. In order to change this, the conscious mind must be activated, and the unconscious mind must be reprogrammed. The man who apparently read up on nutrition and lifestyle had willingly decided to activate the conscious part of his brain in order to make these changes.

Simultaneously, he completed changes that led to repetitive experiences and changes in the unconscious program. His friend was definitely not ready to go outside of her comfort zone. She went into a state of defense and acted out from her preprogrammed unconscious mind.

Up until we are around six or seven years old, the unconscious part of the brain is the active part. With the help of EEG measurements, we can see which type of frequency the brain is operating at.

When we sleep, the brain is operating at *delta* frequencies (0.5–4 Hz). This is an unconscious activity. When we are about to wake up or fall asleep, the brain operates at *theta* frequencies (4–8 Hz). This is the frequency of the brain that operates during imagination, where dreams and reality mix. This frequency is also at play during hypnosis.

When we are going over to an awakened state, the brain works at *alpha* frequencies (8–12 Hz). This is a calm state where we are not completely focused. For example, this can happen when we are on our way to work. When we have reached work, *beta* signals are sent out from the brain. In this state, we are focused and concentrated (12–35 Hz). The last state is when we bring out our peak performance. Now we operate at *gamma* frequencies (>35 Hz).

It is interesting that the brain operates in different frequencies depending on our age. Children up to around one and a half years old operate mostly just in delta mode. This is primarily because the nervous system is poorly developed. An infant's first behavior after birth is a result of inborn reflexes or instincts. Infants have little conscious muscle activity. Input is developed before output. From the ages of around one and a half years old until they are six to seven years old, children operate primarily in theta mode. This is why children have wild imaginations. A child at this age will experience a ride on a broom as riding on a horse. For children, the broom is a real horse. It is interesting that theta mode is used during hypnosis. Hypnosis is a technique to change the subconscious mind. The brain is extremely responsive to instruction and observation. In order to illustrate this stage better, I will use an analogy from everyday life.

Think about when you have just bought a new Apple iPad. You are excited to use it, but before you can, you have to download software. Without software, there is little you can do with an iPad. This is also the case when we are born. We are born with hardware but with limited software.

We use the first six to seven years of life downloading software. We need a database in order to take advantage of the hardware that we were born with. We can also look at the first six to seven years as a video camera where we record events around us, which we later use as a textbook. It is extremely important to remember that what is downloaded in these years is what children observe around them—this means the behavior of the mother, father, siblings, family members, friends, and grown-ups in the kindergarten. This helps to form the unconscious part of the mind 95 percent of our later life is acted from.

The Jesuits had a saying, "Give me the child for the first seven years and I will give you the man." This saying existed long before EEG results were a reality. The saying is probably based on experience. The Jesuits knew that, if they were able to mark the first seven years of a child's life, it would be difficult to break this, since 95 percent of life is controlled by the unconscious mind, which is based on the first six to seven years of life.

The download phase up to six to seven years old is the reason we see characteristics and traits are inherited. It can also be the reason that diseases are inherited. It is not because the traits and diseases are inherited in the genes, but because the genes are programmed by the surroundings. An everyday example is found in the form of phobias and anxiety. There are very few people who have phobias or anxiety based on reality. If you are terrified of thunder and lightning and your child observes your behavior, it is natural that the child will also become scared of thunder and lightning as an adult. Very few people have actually been struck by lightning or have had a physical threatening experience with it. In the same way, very few people who are scared of spiders and snakes have had a threatening experience with any of them. Have you thought about how you express yourself when you speak to children about these animals/insects?

After the age of six to seven years old, the brain begins to operate in alpha mode. This is reflected by children sitting still, being more concentrated, and slowly beginning to learn simple things, without demanding too much of them. This harmonizes very well with starting school. It is worth mentioning that different regions in the brain develop in different sequences and tempos in boys and girls.[45]

The brain is fully developed in men around the age of thirty. However, in women, the brain is fully developed when they are about twenty-two years old. Many women will probably nod and think, *I knew it!*

If we compare how many minutes a thirty-year-old man and a thirty-year-old woman can sit still, be quiet, and pay attention, we would probably not find a big difference. What if we were to compare six-year-olds? On average, how many minutes can a six-year-old boy sit still, be quiet, and pay attention compared to a six-year-old girl? Most teachers will say that boys have bigger problems with this task than do girls. The boys often begin to turn around, fiddle with something, and become restless. Some are even diagnosed with ADHD and medicated. These boys really do not need medicine but a better general understanding that boys and girls develop differently. A normal development and demeanor for a six-year-old girl is not necessarily a normal development for a six-year-old boy. If we would take into consideration how the brain develops, boys should maybe start school later than girls.

There must be harmony between the conscious and the subconscious mind

The conscious part of the mind is creative and can deliberately create positive thoughts. In order for the positive thoughts to have a positive effect, the conscious and unconscious mind must be in harmony. The unconscious mind will automatically limit or sabotage positive thinking if the unconscious mind has a negative experience. If there is conflict between the conscious and the unconscious part of the mind, the unconscious part will always win.

In order to illustrate this, we can observe a child who constantly hears that he or she does not deserve something because he or she is not well behaved or good enough. This will be programmed in the unconscious mind. Remember that this controls 95 percent of our actions in adult life. This programming will sabotage the child for success later on in life. In adult life, this person will feel undeserving of praise, reward, or success because it was not something he or she heard as a child. A consciously positive thought, where you tell yourself that you deserve or will manage to do something, will have little effect if the unconscious mind does not believe in what you are saying.

An important task is to create compliance between belief and reality.

Here's an example. After you have read this book, you decide to make some changes in your life. You wake up, and you are full of enthusiasm. During the day, the unconscious part of the mind takes over, and you respond similarly in the exact same situations as you have done earlier. When you come home, you feel even more sad and frustrated than before you left this morning. You think that life is unfair and, apparently, that you are not meant to be well. You make yourself into a victim, where your fate is predestined based on programs that you have previously downloaded.

Everyday life is full of situations where this principal is applicable, and I'm sure you can think of many examples yourself.

It will not help to tell yourself that today you look damn good if the unconscious mind does not agree. It will be difficult to stop smoking if the unconscious mind does not want to.

In the world of elite sports, this is very apparent. It is difficult to win or become the best if your unconscious mind tells you that others are better. You will lose for sure. Athletes who achieve good results are often "in the zone." Everything you do is successful. You feel invincible. The unconscious mind believes it, and you make yourself into a protein-creating machine made for success.

On the other hand, if the results are absent, negative thoughts will sneak in, and the unconscious mind will gradually begin to believe that you are made for failure. You begin to produce stress hormones, which are created for protection, instead of growth and maintenance. We are not made to be in this state of being over a long period of time. Because of this cascade, the cells are operating in defense mode, you will recover poorly and handle training poorly, and eventually injuries will come.

We will look a little bit closer at research and examples that highlight the importance of compliance between the conscious and unconscious mind and, last but not least, the importance of the mind.

Historically, we can go back to the 1800s and the development of the germ theory. Koch's postulations were not so well accepted by everyone. Since Koch and Pasteur meant *Vibrio cholerae* was the bacterium that was the cause of cholera, a critic wanted to disprove this by drinking a glass containing this bacterium. The man did not become sick.

This attempt has been discussed later on by DiRita, where science dismisses it, claiming that this man was not like everyone else and was not representative.[46] History tells us that this man was so sure that the germ theory was wrong that, without pre-investigation, he drank the poison in order to prove that it was incorrect. There is no doubt that this man's unconscious mind was as convinced as his conscious mind that this theory was not correct.

Another extreme example that there must be compliance between the unconscious and the conscious mind is when a group of people drink poison in deadly doses in order to prove that God is taking care of them.[47]

Walking on burning coals has been practiced for thousands of years. A related record is even registered in *The Guinness Book of World Records* by a twenty-three-year-old Canadian woman. This happened in 2005. The woman walked sixty-seven meters on glowing coal, something that took her thirty seconds.[48] How is it that someone can walk on glowing coal without being hurt, whereas others are severely burned by the exact same coal? This shows how important the brain can be. Simultaneously, it puts a question mark about the materialistic thought process. Quantum physics says that the person who observes has sensory perception and, from this, will create reality (I will come back to this).

There exists an uncountable number of examples of humans who have received a deadly diagnose and have spontaneously recovered and become well again.[49]

There also exist reported cases where normal people lift different vehicles in order to save someone whom they care about after they are stuck in an accident.[50] They are placed in a situation where they have to throw away their limiting beliefs. Remember the importance of the unconscious and the conscious mind agreeing; if not, the unconscious mind will win.[51]

When we use the conscious part of the mind to make a willful action or create a thought, the unconscious part will automatically go into "default." The software that is downloaded into the unconscious part of the mind controls your sensory perception when you think or are in a given situation.

For example, you may love fish for dinner, and today you are invited for fish at a friend's place. Just the thought of it makes you drool. The body gets ready to receive and digest food. The body is in growth and maintenance mode. Switch the scenario. You loathe fish, but today you are invited for fish at your friend's place. You will not make a big scene, and you are trying to convince yourself that the dinner will be okay. Still, when time is getting closer, your mouth will get dry; you will start sweating and feel uncomfortable. Your body is now producing stress hormones designed for fight or flight.

Another example from my own family is when we are in an amusement park with carousels and roller coasters; my daughters love it, but I become nauseous and dizzy as soon as I see a carousel.

Both examples illustrate that two identical situations can provoke different responses depending on how the sensory experience is or how the unconscious mind operates. This brings us to a deeper discussion of perception or sensory experience. The body senses, but the brain interprets what is being sensed.

"Every organ in your body is connected to the one under your hat" (B. J. Palmer, son of D. D. Palmer and founder of chiropractic).

If you have a vision to change the world, your local environment, or your social circle, it is important to begin with yourself. For example, if you are a bad parent, your children will observe you and program this behavior into their unconscious minds. Maybe they will use this program when they become parents and, thus, themselves become bad parents. Characteristics of being a bad parent can, therefore, be passed through generations if one does not change the unconscious program.

I hardly know if I dare to take this further to what is happening in the Middle East. How can we be hopeful of peace when there have been hatred and war between neighbors through generations? Children grow up in the fear of terror and suicide bombs and with a genuine fear that they could lose members of their own family or their own life at any moment. What do you think parents tell their children about their neighbors? Based on what I have discussed earlier in this book, do you think that the children's chemical composition resembles that which belongs to fight or flight or … that which belongs to fight or flight? I can't find room for other alternatives. How do you believe their unconscious mind, which controls 95 percent of who they are, is programmed? Maybe we should think a little bit more about this when refugees arrive. I am aware that this is a big simplification of a very complex situation, but I believe that it brings up a good point nevertheless.

How you perceive will determine your own personal virtual reality

Most of what you perceive as reality is based on what your brain tells you from your sensory perception. Your environment influences your senses and sensations, which is interpreted by the brain.

As I am writing this, I am at my parents' cabin up in the beautiful, wild mountains of Norway. It is early spring. There is no one around, except my dog—all is quiet. There is a small breeze, but it doesn't matter because the sun is heating up the air, and it feels just nice. Crystal blue sky; sunbeams reflected by the snow that will be melted away in a few days; a smell of fresh air, free from pollution; and the view is spectacular, with its tall mountain peaks sunbathing not far away. This is reality—for me. This is how I perceive it.

I wonder, Does my dog perceive it differently? Does she see the beautiful colors? Maybe she is color-blind? I know she hears a lot better than I do (not when I am yelling at her). Maybe she finds the breeze annoying? I am wearing my sunglasses, but I don't have any for her. Maybe she finds the reflecting sunbeams to bright?

Who can tell if my reality is the right reality?

We have no proof that the physical world matches our mental representation of it.

There is no sign of crystal blue in my neurons. There is no breeze in my brain (I hope). My brain has the exact same temperature wherever I am in the world.

Your brain will process the information it receives and produce your own personal virtual reality. The physical reality of an object depends on how you perceive it.

The brain will always adjust itself by the signals from the environment. This is called plasticity. Neuroscience has shown that changes in sensory information lead to a central nervous system that is constantly under reorganization.[52]

It also shows that changes from increased sensory information or decreased sensory information to the brain can lead to changes in structure and function in the nerve cells themselves.[53]

Based on previous experience, learning, and expectations, the brain creates an inner reality based on perception, which does not need to reflect the outer reality. How you respond to your inner reality reflects in your physical actions.

In regards to soccer, I am passionate about my favorite team. It has struck me many times that even a team's own supporters strongly disagree about players' performances after the game. The players are usually evaluated by an "expert", either from their own supporter club or local newspaper and given a grade on a scale from 0 to 10. In the comments section there is usually a strong exchange of opinions about this grading.

A common saying is, "I can't believe we watched the same game!" This illustrates exactly that what we see is not necessarily reflecting reality. Each person can emphasize a different part of the game, such as defensive organization, counter, possession, the result of the match, brilliant individual performances, hard tackling, or full effort. How can half of the spectators at the stadium scream for a penalty while the other half applauds a brilliant tackle?

More scientifically explained, through the view of a child (who is not raised around zebras), a zebra is a horse with stripes. This is called assimilation. They think based on previous experience. Whenever there is strong enough evidence to show that this is not a horse with stripes, but a zebra, the child will recognize this. This is called accommodation. Another example is with shadows.

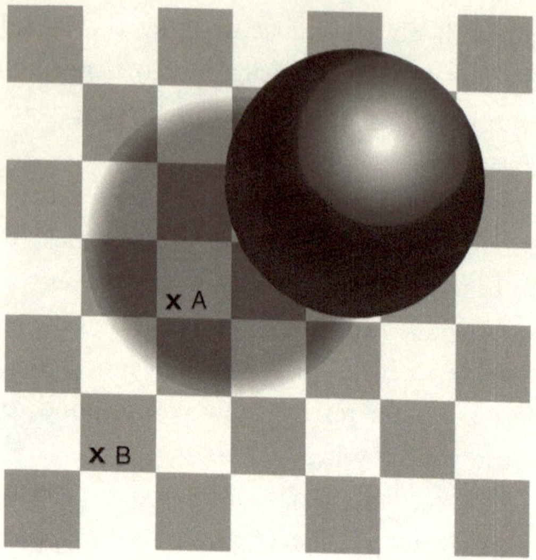

Figure 2.1

You will probably see that the two squares marked with "x" have different shades of gray. This is how the brain interprets this sensory experience from previous experience. If you now cover everything except the two squares marked with "x," you will see they have exactly the same shades of gray.

We have three forms of perception:

1. The instincts, which we are born with (programmed in our genes)
2. Memory from the unconscious part of the brain (especially important during the first seven years of age, since we then operate in theta mode)
3. Action, based on the conscious part of the brain

I have previously concluded that our genetic material does not predetermine our fate, but it is influenced by our sensory experience.

You can do an experiment yourself. If you are able to focus on your own thoughts, it will not take you long.

Sit down in a chair and think about something you are looking forward to, something you like very much, or a situation in the past that you truly appreciated. The body will automatically begin to produce hormones to ensure growth and maintenance. You are in development.

When you have managed to feel that you are truly in the situation, recognize how you feel. Maybe you're smiling, are clear minded, or feeling well balanced.

Sit in the same chair in the same environment and think about something that frightens you—a phobia you have, a fight you had recently, or something similar. When you feel that you are truly in that situation, recognize how you feel now. Do you have clammy hands, an increased heart rate, dilated pupils, and an increased blood pressure? You are in fight-or-flight mode. And if you are here long enough, the body will break down slowly but surely.

Are you a person who becomes irritated when you wait in a grocery line and are frustrated that you always choose the line that goes the slowest? I was. This obviously produced a stress response in my body. I have never documented any specific symptoms, but I assume that I had clammy hands, dilated pupils, increasing blood pressure, an increased heart rate, and reddening in my face. This was not something I wanted but, rather an automatic reaction from my unconscious mind. This changed after I had an interesting conversation with one of my patients. I do not remember how we landed on the topic, but the patient wondered if I, like others, had a busy life. Was it difficult to find time to slow down a little bit? The patient had experienced that standing in line was a superb way to calm down and gather her thoughts. There is not much else to do than to follow the line, so why not use the time for something healthy instead of the exact opposite? After I began to look at it in this manner, my sensory experience of standing in line totally changed. Now I almost look for the longest line or for something to happen that slows down the line so that I have a good reason to calm down without feeling lazy. Now my body can produce the good hormones and ensure growth and development instead of being in fight-or-flight mode.

Here's another example from my own life. Many people—myself included— are taught that sharks are dangerous man-eaters. Very few who have a fear of sharks have had any physical, real experience with them, myself included. In Australia, people have a little more nuanced perception of sharks. While studying in Australia, I had a little bay right next to where I lived. I remember very well one of the first times I snorkeled there. Unexpectedly, I saw a shark. In my opinion, it very much resembled something I had seen in the film *Jaws* (although this one was barely one meter long), and my heart was about to pop out of my chest. I was almost sure that it was going to eat me. I heard the soundtrack from *Jaws* loudly, and I freestyle stroked in the best Disney style in order to come out of the water as fast as possible. I was shaking for a while after I reached the shore. On the way back on a popular footpath along this bay, I suddenly heard someone scream, "Shark!" The funny thing was that instead of people swimming toward the shore and getting out of the water, which I had expected, there were many who jumped in and swam toward the person who screamed shark. They also wanted to have a look!

After a while, it became known to me that there were seven dusky whaler sharks that had residence in this bay. These are harmless sharks and don't have humans on their menu. Subsequently, I spent a lot of time around these sharks. Eventually, I knew these sharks so well that I gave them different names based on their character traits.

Today, I think sharks are fascinating, and I have swum together with them on various occasions. Practically, this means that I have reprogrammed the unconscious part of my mind in regards to my perception of sharks. Previously, adrenaline was circulating in my body and my fight-or-flight response was working to its fullest capacity when I saw or thought about a shark. This is proof that the same perception can lead to radical opposites in terms of how the body reacts based on what is programmed in the unconscious part of the mind, whether the situation is actual or thought based. It also illustrates that it is possible to reprogram the unconscious part of the mind you instinctively act upon. After getting information about these dusky whaler sharks and, eventually, having positive experiences, I used the conscious part of my mind to change the unconscious part.

These simple examples illustrate three important aspects:

1. Your sensory experience controls which adequate responses your body will give.
2. The body will react in an approximately similar way, independent of whether you are in a real situation or if you just think that you're in that situation.
3. You can actively take part in influencing your fate.

Our sensory experience influences life already before conception. A study shows that a mother's and father's state of mind before conception influences the quality of sperm and egg cells. If you find yourself in a phase of life before conception where the body is mostly in protection mode and has less energy for growth and maintenance, this can lead to poor quality of the sperm cells and egg cells. The contents within a mother's blood crosses into the placenta. It is not just nutrients from a mother that is transported over to the fetus, but also the different signals that a state of mind produces. If the mother is happy and satisfied, that state will produce a fetus with the same good hormones. If the mother is stressed, stress hormones will cross into the placenta, and the child's cells will receive a notice to protect itself and not grow and develop in the way that it should. The fetus will already begin to "observe" its environment and, thus, begin the programming of the unconscious part of the mind.

Placebo: Yes, please

This brings us to the placebo effect. The placebo effect can influence both the body and the mind. It can give side effects (nocebo) and desired effects. It can make symptoms arise, and it can make them disappear. The placebo effect changes people's lives.

The placebo effect can be defined as how belief and values form the brain's function in relation to perception and feelings and mental and physical health.[54]

Every medical treatment is surrounded by a psychosocial context, which influences the therapeutic outcome. If we study the psychosocial context, we must eliminate the real effect of the treatment and simulate a context, which is similar to that which occurs during treatment and in reality. A fake treatment is given without the test subjects knowing, so that the test subjects believe the treatment is effective and expect improvements. The placebo effect is the effect we receive after a fake treatment. Insight into the placebo effect is insight into the psychosocial context around the patient.

There are different types of placebo effects. The most common explanation is found in classical conditioning and expectation. A lot of research conducted around the placebo effect up until today is about RCT (randomized controlled trials), with roots in allopathic medicine. It means that most of the studies in this area concern pain or analgesia. More recently, many studies have been conducted on the placebo effect in relation to other things, like the immune system, motor disorders, and depression. Psychosocial studies, studies of behavior, and diagnostic imaging have contributed to our acceptance of the placebo effect today. The overview over the placebo effect has developed into a good model in order to understand how complex mental activity, for example expectation, influences the nervous system.[55]

Some believe that the placebo effect always is a contributory cause of an effect based on an intervention. Others believe that it is meaningless.[56]

In a study published by the *Journal of Clinical Psychology*, 2007, researchers analyzed how many patients must be treated in order to get an effect from placebo and how many more were needed in order to get an effect from a special treatment.[57] Lower amounts have larger effects. In comparison to those not receiving any treatment at all, 7 patients were needed to reach the effect of 1, in relation to the placebo. In addition, 8 patients were required in order to achieve the effect of 1 person regarding radiotherapy for breast cancer. The amount is 24 for beta-blockers for chronic heart failure, 12 for influenza vaccine, and 208 for preventative treatment with aspirin for heart attack.

The fact that different studies give contradictory results when analyzed should, on its own, be an indication of the placebo effect. One finds what one is looking for, or one achieves the effect one believes one will achieve. It is fascinating that one can almost guess who the author of a study is just by seeing the conclusion of the study.

Having said that, this also applies to myself. My opinions are formed from previous experiences, belief, and feelings.

The relationship between the practitioner and the patient; the patient's expectations, desires and needs, personality, and degree of discomfort from the symptoms; and the environment are all examples of factors that play a part in the placebo effect.

Based on my understanding, I will give some examples of how I believe the placebo effect can unfold in my clinical practice.

When I sit down with a patient for the first time, it is not uncommon that the patient says, "Typical, today when I'm finally going to do something about this problem, it is not so bad." Many will, as a matter of fact, experience an improvement after they have made the initial appointment. The explanation lies in the placebo effect. Unfortunately, we have been taught that, when something does not feel right, we have to go to the doctor. This point of view has arisen following the mechanistic, reductionist, and deterministic thought process highlighted earlier in the book. Since this thought process is based on disease, misery, bad genes, bad luck, bacteria, and virus, there is not anything you can do yourself but seek help.

This is a smart move in order to make us dependent on help from the outside.

Think back to your childhood or what you say to your children when they have a fever, are coughing, or have a headache or bad rash. They have to go to the doctor, and eventually they will need medicine. As long as this is programmed into your unconscious mind, that is what you expect. When you pick up the telephone and call your doctor or, in this instance, me, the chiropractor, you will begin to feel better because you have now started a process you believe will make you feel better. Your body will begin to produce other hormones, which lead to a changed inner chemical composition. This part of the placebo effect can be seen in context to classical conditioning. You associate a previous happening with a physiological change because you have experienced it so many times.

If you have had a headache many times and experienced that it disappears with the use of painkillers, you will automatically seek the external help of painkillers in order to help your inner state when you experience headaches. Every time this happens, it will create an associated learning, and the effect will become stronger because it created a network of nerve cells, where nerve cells are activated simultaneously. A well-known expression in neuroscience is "nerve cells that fire together, wire together" (Hebb's law). After a while, you would probably receive the same effect from a sugar pill as you do from a real painkiller pill.

Another example from my everyday practice is that it is much easier to achieve good results with those patients who consult me because they have heard good things about me or were recommended to visit me by someone who is or has been satisfied with my service than with those who feel compelled to consult me. I also believe that this is related to the placebo effect. I will later refer to some scientific studies that support that optimism and positivity lead to improvement.

A third example from my own practice is that it is also easier to achieve good results with those who truly need good results. That can include patients in severe pain. It can be patients who have to become better quickly because they have something they want to be a part of in the immediate future, requiring them to be in good shape. It can also be patients who are financially limited. They simply cannot afford treatment, but at the same time, they do not want discomfort. They just have to get better with as little help as possible. They will do whatever I tell them to do on their own.

A fourth example from my practice is when I adjust a patient, a cavitation or a cracking sound will most likely happen. Many patients associate this sound with chiropractic. Many patients can become excited, anxious, curious, and full of expectations when hearing such cracking sounds. The patient themselves will both hear and feel a specific adjustment. It is not always that there is a need for an adjustment that produces a sound, and it is not always that I manage exactly what I intended either. If the patient expects a cavitation, and it does not happen, I have experienced that this can lead to poorer results. If both the patient and I expect a cavitation, but it is absent because I didn't achieve the intention, I experience that the effect may become reduced.

My second, third, and fourth examples can all be explained by expectation, which is one of the elements regarding the placebo effect. In our mind, we envision and expect a better future. If the body's feelings comply with what we expect, we will not be able to distinguish between expected improvements and actual improvement.

When a cracking sound creates an expectation and a placebo effect, just think about the expectations and faith that underlie a heart surgery, where the surgical team splits the sternum and opens the thorax in order to gain access to the heart, or aggressive chemotherapy and radiotherapy. Do you think that the placebo effect could be a part of the reason one becomes better?

I believe that the placebo effect is extremely undervalued and misunderstood. Unfortunately, as it is today, for most people in the evidence-based group, the placebo is nothing more than another technical term that is taken advantage of in order to evaluate whether a physically measurable measure helps or not. Because the placebo is looked upon as a fake measure, treatment measures where placebo is the contributory factor is considered cheating or trickery. The placebo effect is, in the highest degree, an effect and when we separate placebo from nocebo (a non-desired effect), it is also a desired effect.

When the principle "primum non nocere" (do no harm) is taken into consideration, a desired effect is exactly what a practitioner should be interested in achieving. If I find placebo as an effect because someone believes or expects a certain outcome, I would like to have as much help as possible from the placebo effect when I deal with my patients. It is not that I do not have confidence in chiropractic as a method of treatment, but I am all for the expression, "Yes, both please." The fact that the placebo effect apparently has an effect makes me interested in knowing more about the brain's influence on the body, so that I can help my patients in an effective and gentle way.

I spend a lot of time together with my patients during the first two consultations. The first consultation consists of a thorough history of my patient's health and an examination in order to collect relevant information and assess the condition of the patient. The second consultation, in large part, is used to explain findings and try to place the findings in context with how the patient feels. I emphasize that there will be compliance between the findings, advice, and care plan. It is important to speak in a language that the patient understands. The better the patient understands my "educated guesses," the greater the placebo effect will be and the greater the implementation will be. After close to 100,000 consultations, I can often tell the patient, as a result of the examination, what kind of symptoms I expect they have. If I ask/tell them, without the patient telling me, there will be an even greater chance for the placebo effect if my expectation is right.

The same applies for the plan. If I manage to make a plan that complies with how the patient feels, this will reinforce the placebo effect. If I tell the patient that my expectation is that the symptoms should subside after five treatments and the patient is still in pain, the placebo effect will be reduced. This is one of the hardest things to decide as a practitioner because everyone responds differently. I would like the patient to become well as quickly as possible, but if I give an estimate that doesn't hold up, this can strike back on the treatment effect. This also applies the other way. If the patient is told that they will become better in twelve weeks, there is little probability that it will take six weeks (less time). Especially within sports medicine, I believe that it is a challenge that all injuries are estimated to time. I believe that this creates a limitation on the course of treatment. In my own practice, I'd rather try to set a plan based on function rather than time. When an objective is reached, we can go further to the next objective.

I think that the placebo effect as a phenomenon is not interesting enough to conventional medicine or business owners because it is free of charge and occurs on the body's premises. No profit, no interest. If we can create desired effects with our own minds, to me, this is exceptionally interesting.

When patients have attempted alternative treatment, they often tend to hold back and are embarrassed to tell me about it. When I attempt to help a patient, I will always want to know what has made them better and what has made them worse. Whether it is chiropractic, acupuncture, osteopathy, reflexology, faith healing, hypnotherapy, or crystals, I find it interesting as long as the treatment has had an effect, which has not caused the patient any harm. My job is to try to understand these effects in order to integrate or develop my own philosophy and treatment simultaneously, as the main principle, primum non nocere (do no harm), remains unchanged. It is not always easy to know whether the effect is just caused by the mind or the mind due to the body. We must remember that all effects are related to the mind, since the brain interprets the signals of the body.

We will now look a little bit closer at the scientific documentation behind the placebo effect.

Several hundred thousand patients every year have surgery for osteoarthritis in the knee by the help of arthroscopy. This is a method (called arthroscopy) where a small incision is made, whereupon a little fiber-optic instrument is led into the joint so that the surgeon can see how the joint looks from the inside. The surgeon will scrape and rinse out the degenerated cartilage, which is believed to be the cause of the patient's pain and discomfort. It is still uncertain why many patients become better from this treatment. In 1996, the American Orthopedic surgeon Bruce Moseley conducted, with several others, a study that considered whether the placebo effect is a part of the cause for the results.[58]

Five test subjects were randomly picked out to be in the placebo group. This group received a small incision in the knee. They were sown up without further treatment. Three test subjects were randomly picked to be in a group that would be operated with a procedure that is called lavage. This procedure consists of high-pressured water that is inserted in the joint in order to clean and rinse away the damaged tissue. Two test subjects were randomly picked out for a standard arthroscopy procedure, where the surgeon removes unwanted cartilage. All of the procedures were conducted under anesthesia. Dr. Moseley, who conducted the surgery, was also himself unaware (blinded) during and after the surgery, which patient he was operating on, by drawing an envelope that told him what type of procedure would be conducted.

After the surgery, all of the test subjects reported that they had better mobility and less pain. After six months, there was no difference between the test subjects. After six years, two test subjects from the placebo group still said that they walked normally, without pain and with better mobility. These test subjects felt that they received their lives back after the placebo surgery. This was a small pilot study. The conclusion was that more studies should be conducted in order to ascertain the placebo effect.

This was also done. In 2002, Dr. Moseley published a new study in *The New England Journal of Medicine* with 180 patients.[59]

This study showed the same results as the pilot study. Patients in all of the three groups experienced improved health after the surgery. Neither of the two groups who received the actual surgery achieved better results than the placebo group. The same applied two years later.

In December 2013, a Finish study was published in *The New England Journal of Medicine* regarding arthroscopic meniscectomy.[60]

The test subjects had torn the medial (inner) meniscus. The study design was double-blinded RCT. A total of 146 test subjects participated in the study. An inclusion criterion was that the test subjects could not have osteoarthritis in the same knee as the meniscus injury.

This study concluded, similarly to the two previous studies, that those who were operated on did not become any better than those who were not operated on. The results were still similar after two years.

Lars Engebretsen, professor and research director at the orthopedic center at Oslo University Hospital, Ullevål and professor at the Center for Sport Injury Research at Norway's Sport College, said on October 1, 2014, to *Dagens Medisin*, "General practitioners must learn that patients with worn meniscus should not be operated on and the orthopedic surgeons have to stop operating on them."

Can it be that these patients become better simply because they believe that they will be better? Is the belief reinforced at the hospital, with medical personnel in coats, face masks, and hats and the fact that the body is being cut into? If this is the case, how do you think the belief in improvement becomes if we talk about a more comprehensive heart surgery, where the entire sternum (breastbone) would be split open? I think a very strong belief and confidence are needed to become a part of this. We must remember that there does not exist any RCT studies that say anything about the effect of these types of surgery. We have only empirical evidence and explanations based on anatomical and physiological knowledge.

Available data from experimental studies show that the placebo effect influences a range of autonomous functions.

Studies show the placebo effect influences the immune system, gastrointestinal activity and the length of the stomach's contraction periods, the respiratory system, and the cardiovascular system.[61]

Studies also show how the placebo effect influences different areas in the brain.[62] Diagnostic imaging can show the influence of the neurochemical function.[63]

Oxytocin is a neuropeptide that is released when we have positive feelings. Oxytocin closes the receptors in a center of the brain called the amygdala. The amygdala is the part of the brain that activates fear and distress. With fear and distress out of the way, it will again be easier to create positive feelings, which ensures the further production of oxytocin. Oxytocin also has a healing effect on a number of organs. Later studies show that the receptors in the intestines, immune system, liver, heart, and other organs respond to oxytocin. Examples of these effects are the regulation of blood sugar, blood vessels in the heart, better gastrointestinal function, and stimulation of the immune system. [64]

A range of studies shows that what we think and how we feel influences our health. In 2000, the Mayo Clinic published a study where 839 people were followed over a thirty-year period in order to see if optimists had higher survival rates than pessimists.[65] The study concluded that pessimists are associated with a significantly increased likelihood of early death.

In 2002, the Mayo Clinic published a similar study, where researchers followed 447 people for more than thirty years.[66] The study showed that optimists had both better physical and better mental health than did pessimists.

In addition, other studies show that optimism influences our health.[67]

A study from Yale, published in the same year, concluded that people with a positive demeanor toward becoming old lived more than seven years longer than those who are negative.[68] A study from the University of North Carolina showed that positive feelings increased the activity in the vagal nerve, which plays a central role in the regulation of the autonomous nervous system and our homeostasis.[69]

Placebo is more effective than antidepressants. In 1998, the psychologist Irving Kirsch, PhD, published a meta-analysis of published RCTs of antidepressants.[70] Out of nineteen studies with 2,318 patients, most of the results were due to the placebo effect, not the effect of medicine. The correlation between the placebo effect and the effect of medicine was recorded to be as high as 0.9. This study attracted attention and made many people keep their eyes open for the placebo effect.

In 2008, Kirsch published a new study that considered the placebo effect against the effect of four of the most prescribed antidepressants.[71] The study looked at thirty-five RCTs from 1987 until 1999 with more than 5,000 patients. The study concluded that, even here, a difference in the effect of the most frequently prescribed medicines and the placebo effect does not exist.

It is worth noting that none of these studies proves that antidepressants do not work; on the contrary, they do work, but not better than placebo.

There exists a range of other studies looking at the context between the effect of antidepressants and the placebo effect.[72]

From a medical perspective, it is suggested that it is no longer necessary to make several placebo-controlled studies in order to test out new alternative treatments, since there already exists many studies that show the effect of medicine when it comes to depression![73]

Significant evidence of the placebo response in scientific studies of antidepressants has further justified studies within this area.[74]

It has been shown that the placebo effect can arise by the observation of others in a social context, without any further reinforcement from the observer. Colloca and Bendetti published a study in 2009, where they looked at the pain relief the placebo effect gave off to observe someone who simulated a pain-relieving effect. The effect achieved was equally as strong as that for the one who received the actual pain-relieving medicine. The study also showed that stronger empathy leads to a stronger placebo response.[75]

In 2010, a surprising study was published that showed that the placebo effect was present even when the test subjects knew that they received the placebo as an intervention.[76]

The study contained forty test subjects with an irritable gastrointestinal tract who were informed that they had received placebo pills. Simultaneously, they were informed that the placebo effect in itself could lead to improvements of symptoms. A control group containing forty other test subjects received no treatment at all. After three weeks, the group that knew about the placebo pills reported double the relief of symptoms as compared to the control group. This result diverts from the previous belief that the placebo effect was dependent on one not knowing the type of intervention administered.

Based on a range of studies, of which some are presented here, it is apparent that the placebo effect plays an important role in the outcome of treatment. A study by Colloca among others in 2004 shows that treatments where the patient knows what is going on and expects improved health is more effective than hidden treatment, where the patient doesn't know anything and doesn't expect a change.[77]

In the same way, an expected medical intervention has a stronger effect than a medical intervention that is unexpected.[78]

These findings show that the effect of medicine is reduced if there does not exist an expectation of its effectiveness, while simultaneously emphasizing that the expectation of the treatment's effect in itself is important to the outcome.

In another study, researchers noticed twice as good effects when patients were informed when the painkillers were given, as supposed to not being informed. Furthermore, this study showed that, when test subjects were told that the medicine was no longer being given, it led to reduced pain relief with associated changes in the brain, even though the medicine was still being given.[79]

These findings indicate that expectation has a strong influence on the response from painkiller medicine. The study shows that even the placebo effect when it comes to painkiller medicine is reversible.

Nocebo

In Latin, *nocebo* means, "I will harm," in contrast to *placebo*, which means, "I will please." The concept of nocebo was introduced into our modern lexicon in order to describe the negative effects of placebo.[80] Today, nocebo refers to something that causes a harmful effect, based on negative expectations.

In 1962, a study was conducted in Japan that illustrates the nocebo effect.[81] The test subjects were thirteen children who were extremely allergic to a poisonous plant. A harmless leaf was rubbed on one of the child's arms as the child was told that this plant was poisonous. On the other arm, a leaf from the poisonous plant was rubbed, and the children were told that it was not harmless. All of the children developed a rash on the arm that was rubbed with the harmless leaf, which they believed to be poisonous. Eleven of the thirteen children didn't develop a rash on the arm exposed to the poison, but which they thought was harmless.

In this instance, the belief that the leaf was harmless was greater than what the body remembered from experience. In the second instance, a harmless leaf became harmful, simply because of the belief that it was harmful. The study shows in both instances that the mind plays an important role in our health.

Due to ethical issues, there exist relatively few studies on the nocebo effect. The studies that have been conducted previously had, in a large part, healthy volunteers who received verbal stimulus.[82]

The body and mind cannot be separated

Since the placebo effect is demonstrably a real neurobiological phenomenon that is meaningful in neuroscience and health care, we should spend more effort to find out how we will use this phenomenon in a clinical setting. The placebo effect is not limited to an artificial placebo intervention in double-blinded RCTs. The placebo effect's existence shows that we should expand our horizons and let go of our limiting beliefs of our human possibilities.

When you see how strong the influence of belief and feelings are, how does it influence your everyday life? Do you think all the death and misery that is reported in the news influences you? Do the health authorities influence you when they warn about the influenza season and recommend that you pay your doctor a visit to get your annual influenza shot? Do you think that the commercials on TV about painkiller medicine, nasal spray, and cough syrup influence you? As a practicing therapist, I often hear from my patients that their condition is certainly due to age, and there is nothing to do about it. Is this simply because we are bombarded with information about the normality of stiffer joints, blood pressure medicine, cholesterol medicine, less energy, bad memory and a reduced sexual drive when we grow older?

I will also put a big question mark on taking advantage of double-blinded RCT as the methodical gold standard, since placebo apparently has its effect. In my opinion, there is no doubt that the mind is deceptive. Your interpretation of the surroundings controls your inner reality. I believe that serious fallacies are made when this aspect is excluded. As we will see in this book, I put a big question mark on the scientific truths that are exclusively based on such studies. The placebo phenomenon should lead to a change in study design and clinical attempts that can be applied to a patient-practitioner interaction.

In *Healing from Within*, Dennis T. Jaffe, PhD, wrote:

The patient must be guided toward discovering the healing powers that lie within him. Faith in pills and external treatments can be replaced by faith in oneself. How would you react upon learning that you have a life-threatening illness? Most people initially sink into a state of anger and despair. They cry, "Why me?" as a protest against the seeming injustice of it all. Physicians find it difficult to answer this desperate question—for example, in grade school we learn the truism that disease is caused by germs. We assume that when a virus or a bacterium hits us, we will get sick, unless we have been vaccinated against it. With this defensive attitude that externals are to blame for illness, it is no wonder that many individuals are chronically worried about their health. If people believe they live in a germ-filled, polluted environment and that they are weak because of inherited psychological and physiological deficiencies, they will perceive themselves as helpless and victimized when they become ill.[83]

In the words of C. S. Gonstead, DC, "The best immune system is in the body, not in Lab."

By the help of neuroscience and physiological approaches, we have a good overview of complex mental factors such as the placebo effect and the relationship between the practitioner and the patient. There should be strong enough evidence to realize that the body and mind is one and that biology and psychology cannot be separated.

If thought alone can change our physiology, we should focus more on which thoughts we think.

We think about sixty thousand to seventy thousand thoughts per day. Around 90 percent of these thoughts are the same as those we had the day before.

These same thoughts lead us to take the same choices and will develop into habits. These habits cause us to experience the same events, which produce the same feelings, which again contribute to producing the same thoughts. When thoughts create a feeling and the feeling creates a thought based on this feeling, you have entered into a circle in which you stay the way you are. Nothing changes.

The biological explanation is that the same thought activates the same nerve signals in the brain, which leads to the same inner chemical composition, signaling to the same genes in the same way and producing the same proteins, allowing us to stay the way we are.

Neuroscience today, calls it identity.

In this circle, your future is predetermined by your past.

Your personality is defined by how you think, how you act, and how you feel.

As Joe Dispenza says, "You are the placebo"; your personality creates your personal reality.

What happens when we break out of this circle?

A new thought will lead to another decision. Another decision leads to another behavior. A new behavior leads to new feelings. New feelings lead to new thoughts.

In other words, a new thought leads to the activation of other nerve signals. Other nerve signals lead to another inner chemical composition. Another inner chemical composition gives other messages to the genes to produce other proteins. You have changed!

When the same genes are still activated by the same signals from the brain, the body will eventually create proteins of poor quality. We become sick, and the body ages. This is what is happening to our skin when we become older. It becomes thinner, and we develop wrinkles because we can no longer produce proteins of the same good quality as before.

Quantum Physics

Create your own future

The brain is involved in everything that makes you who you are, including how you think, feel, and behave. The brain is the organ that constitutes your personality, your intelligence, and your decision-making abilities.

If you have a well-functioning brain, you will most likely have better health, be smarter and happier, make better choices, and probably live longer.

In order to have a well-functioning brain, it is important to give it the right stimulus, like proper nutrition; physical activity; and, last but not least, healthy thoughts.

We will look a little bit closer at how parts of the brain work and how we can actively be a part in creating changes in our future.

I will now talk about things based on quantum mechanics and consequences of Einstein's theory of relativity. This concerns invisible energies instead of matter, and it will appear as abstract in relation to Newton's laws. I hope you will come along on a little journey to the land of opportunities.

"The real voyage of discovery consists not in seeking new landscapes but in having new eyes" (Marcel Proust).

The beginning of the end for Newton's laws

Descartes was the predecessor of the materialistic viewpoint that many still have today. He thought physical and predictable laws controlled the universe. With these laws, Descartes bumped into a problem. Human thoughts have too many variables to fit into these predictable laws. Descartes solved this problem by claiming that the laws that applied to the objective physical world did not apply to the mind. The mind was being held outside of the scientific realm and belonged to the religious realm instead.

Two thousand years after Newton, Einstein developed his theory of relativity and the well-known mass energy law, E=mc2. It shows that energy and matter is one and the same. In order for the acceptance of the theory of relativity, many of the approved nineteenth-century truths had to be rejected. The universal validity of Newton's view about absolute time and space had to be rejected.

An atom is 99.99999 percent energy and only .00001 percent matter. Earlier in the book we have seen that the atom is not the smallest particle there is. It is also an established viewpoint that atoms are not made of matter, but of energy.

We can't explain how a digital watch operates by studying its parts, because a digital watch originates from quantum mechanics and functions as energy in movement. The reductionist approach, with focus on the individual material parts, cannot explain the functions and events in a quantum universe.

Everything physical that you observe is not tangible matter but mostly energy. If we have this as a basic premise, it is ironic that we continue to direct all of our attention to the material aspect when trying to understand reality.

It is claimed that we express just 1.5 percent of our DNA, while the other 98.5 percent lies dormant and waits to be used.

Electrons can exist simultaneously in infinite possibilities in an invisible energy field. The wave-particle duality says that quantum mechanical particles can behave differently. Sometimes, they behave as a wave (energy). For example, this happens when they break around a corner or as the wave phenomenon called interference. Other times they behave as a particle (physical particle), where it is possible to measure an electron's position.

A quantum experiment can prove that electrons can exist simultaneously in an infinite amount of possibilities in an invisible energy field. The particle does not need to define its state until the moment one measures it. The particle is in superposition. When a particle is not in a defined state, we must work with expected values.

It is only when an observer focuses the attention toward an electron that the electron can turn to its defined state. Practically speaking, an electron that behaves as a wave will collapse when it is observed. Quantum physicists call this "the observer effect." Explained in a different way, if you already see a desired event in the future based on your personal wishes, this event already exists in the quantum field. It is just waiting for you to observe it.

Think about using your conscious mind to decide what will become your reality! You can create your own future! Stay with me.

Thoughts and feelings

Think about your love for chocolate. Recently, you have gained about one or two kilograms. You have decided that you will not eat chocolate for a while. A few days later, you are sitting at home and you are bored. You know that you have a bag of M&Ms lying in the cupboard. You notice your body screaming for M&Ms. You think that it can't hurt to have just a few … and, whoops, the bag is empty! Your body's feelings took control over the thought you had about losing weight. Your conscious mind plays the second fiddle.

We communicate with the quantum field through our thoughts and feelings. We can think about it as thoughts being the brain's language and feelings being the body's language. Thoughts and feelings behave like waves. If they are not coordinated, they will offset one another, and we will receive no effect.

I am sure that you can find many examples from your everyday life where you have experienced a desire leading to failure because your feelings did not believe your thoughts.

An experiment from Heart Math Research Center, shows how our thoughts and feelings influence matter (in this experiment, DNA).[84] The experiment also demonstrates that the quantum field does not respond to our wishes or thoughts separately, but when these two are coordinated, they send out similar signals.

Think of thoughts as electric signals that are sent out into the quantum field, whereas feelings are magnetic charges. The thoughts that we think send out an electric signal to the field, whereas our feelings attract the events back to us.

Think about when you have experienced something that made you feel sorry for yourself. Your thoughts will send out signals that are equal to you feeling sorry for yourself. If your feelings are in compliance with your thoughts, your feelings will attract an event that complies with these frequencies and give you a good reason to feel sorry for yourself. Do you recognize the statement, "Why does this always happen to me"? You have probably asked for it.

As long as you follow the same routines, think the same thoughts, and have the same feelings, you will have the same electromagnetic signature, and you will create the same reality. If you are to achieve change, you must think, feel, and act in a different way.

Many people give up when they have been sick or have had problems over a long period of time. They have tried "everything" when it comes to treatment in order to become better, without any success. Bad familiar feeling lead to the same negative thoughts, which lead to the same actions (bad habits), leading further to one hanging on to the past. Some will now look for something completely different and begin to trust the placebo effect or the mind at work. Maybe that is not such a bad decision after all. In order for the placebo effect to work, it requires you to think better thoughts than you feel. When you think new healthy thoughts, this will lead to feeling differently, which again will stimulate more good thoughts. The end product is a change for the better. This is an example of how the placebo effect (or the mind) can be extremely effective.

We have until now established that we are 99.99999 percent energy and .00001 percent matter. This energy behaves like small minitornadoes with infinite possibilities, independent of time and place. It is only by observation, which can be yours, that energy collapses into a particle and appears as a reality, where you can, in compliance with thoughts and feelings, create your own future.

There is no doubt the subjective mind has an effect on the objective world. By thinking the same thoughts and feeling the same feelings, you will continue to create the same events in your life, leading to experiencing the same feelings and thinking similarly in regards to these feelings. You have entered into a bad circle. If you think and feel in a similar way as your environment, you will just confirm your reality and create more of the same.

In order to make a change, you have to think independently of the environment, body, and time.

Free Yourself from the Environment, Body, and Time

Free yourself from the environment

Everything that we have been exposed to during our lives has been saved in the brain as synaptic connections. We can see this in regards to our memory. When we are in the same situations, the brain will remember. The transmission of signals is more effective and will produce the same feelings and thoughts as before. Hebb's law says, "Nerve cells that fire together, wire together." These synaptic connections become more effective by repetition and stronger stimulus, for example a trauma.[85] New connections can be created, old ones can be eliminated, and connections can be strengthened or weakened. The more these networks of neurons are activated, the more apparent they become. Over time, they will develop into an unconscious habit.

These networks that are created in the brain constitute your personality. On the flipside, we can see that your personality controls your personal reality.

In your everyday routine, you wake up at the same time, get ready in the same order, drink coffee out of your favorite coffee mug, and eat the same breakfasts from the same bowl. Then you drive the same way to work, you listen to the same radio station, you see the same people at work, and you hurry home in order to eat dinner at your usual seat by the dinner table. You have to do this before you walk your dog in the usual way, see the same TV show, and go to sleep on the same side of the bed in order to do the same thing again the next day. In this circle, you are confined to reproducing the same experiences that will not provide any changes in your life. Routines make the same signals go to the same genes and lead to the production of the same proteins over and over again. This leads to proteins with bad quality, sickness, and probably an earlier death!

You are not caught up in this bad circle because you have been unfortunate or life is unfair. You have created this circle yourself, and only you can get yourself out of it.

Our brain is mostly a reflection of our past and our surroundings. Because our surroundings, with all of their problems and unwanted situations, control how you think and feel, life is controlled by the surroundings.

When you think based on previous experiences, you can only re-create earlier events. If you re-create the same events, the brain will most likely think and feel the way you are used to thinking and feeling and continue to confirm life the way that you recognize it. Since the brain is a reflection of your surroundings, you will live in the same reality.

Albert Einstein defined madness as doing the same thing over and over again in the hope of a different result. Why are so many people hoping for change, when they think the same thoughts every day, do the same routines, and experience the same feelings? By using the principles of quantum physics, you are now able to understand why this is madness. The science about the nervous system has proven that, by just changing your thoughts, you can change your belief, attitude, actions, and thus your brain.[86]

If you manage to believe in a future you cannot see or experience, and you have thought it so many times that your feelings comply with your thoughts, and you live as if your desired future has already happened, then the brain is no longer a history of your past but a map of your future!

Free yourself from the body

Your five classic senses (touch, smell, hear, see, and taste) will give you a variety of experiences.

When new sensory information reaches the brain, neurons will organize special networks and produce a chemical signal. This is called a feeling or an emotion. Feelings are the result of previous experiences.

When these signals reach the body, you will feel an inner change where you think and feel differently than before you had the sensory experience. When you can recognize what in your environment led to a concrete inner state, you have created a memory.

One example is when you have a bad day. You are caught up in situations that fires up the same signals. You are living in the past because your body thinks that it is experiencing the same situation repeatedly.

To learn is to create new synapses in the brain.

Every day when you have a thought, a biochemical reaction occurs in the brain that produces ligands. These neurotransmitters, neuropeptides, or hormones are created in different parts of the brain and have different mechanisms of action. When the body receives the signals, the body starts up a response that adjusts to the signals that are being created when you think this particular thought. The body sends a message back to the brain telling the brain that it feels the same way the brain is thinking.

Remember that thoughts are the brain's language, and feelings are the body's language. The brain registers how the body feels all the time. It will produce different chemical signals based on feelings from the body. We begin to feel how we think and then think how we feel. When feelings control how we think or we cannot think better thoughts than the way we feel, we get stuck.

Change requires that we think better thoughts and act better than how we feel.

You have probably experienced a blackout when you were trying to remember your PIN code for your credit card. When you reached the cashier or ATM, your fingers were still able to type in the correct code. You didn't manage to consciously remember the code, but your unconscious mind had typed the code so many times that the body remembered it. This is an example of the body controlling the brain, not the opposite.

Think about when you have felt awful for a while. The body has sent out crappy feelings, and your brain has responded by thinking thoughts that are in compliance with how you feel. This cycle is repeated countless times, and you have eventually created a new network in the brain, which makes it even easier to activate this state when the body feels awful. The body simply controls who you are. In quantum physics, the brain is the boss, and the body is the brain's servant, who always obeys. In the example above, the servant has become the boss.

Habits are unconscious actions where the unconscious mind signals to the body. When the body remembers better than the conscious mind, the body has taken the brain's function. Now the body controls the outcome. Conscious positive thoughts always lose to unconscious negative thoughts.

The body behaves quite similarly when it comes to dependence on feelings and intoxicating agents. In the beginning, it takes only a little in order to get a reaction. Eventually, the cells need more and more in order to receive the same response. When the body has become the boss over the brain, it is similar to being in rehab if you want to change yourself.

Most of us live in the past. We have become dependent on the same familiar feelings because the body has memorized our inner chemical states, which are connected to previous events. If we consciously want a better future, we will have to hold back the body's unconscious feelings.

We send new signals to the brain that produce new proteins by changing how we think, feel, and behave. A cell can create thousands of variations from the same genes, without a change in the DNA code. This means that we can send signals to our genes so that we can influence our own future.

A study from Japan shows how happiness can change the genetic expression.[87] People dependent on insulin with type 2 diabetes were divided into two different groups. One group saw a comedy for one hour before they ate a large meal, whereas the other group witnessed a boring, lengthy lecture. The group that saw the lecture had an average increase in blood sugar level by 123 mg/dl, something that equals the need for insulin in order to avoid staying in the danger zone. The other group, who saw a comedy, recorded only half of the rise in blood sugar as the other group. This is only a little over what is normal after a large meal. In addition, the group that saw a comedy changed twenty-three different genetic expressions.

When we think and feel the same way for the most part of our life, our inner state will activate the same genes repeatedly and create the same proteins repeatedly. The body is not an eternity machine. If we activate the same gene sequences all the time, the body will eventually begin to produce proteins of poorer quality. As previously mentioned, this occurs during development of wrinkles. The body produces collagen and elastin of poorer quality. This is also the reason that change is important. Habits make us hold a steady course toward our genetic fate.

Free yourself from time

In the present, all possibilities exist independent of time and place. The opportunities wait to be observed so that waves (energy) collapse into particles (matter). We are not "human beings" but "humans becoming." If we live in the past, none of these potentials gets the chance to be expressed. Living in the past would be letting the body and your environment control your life.

Traumatic events have a tendency to "get stuck" in the brain. This means that the brain produces stronger connections that can be easily reproduced by unconscious stimuli, which has similarity traits with the traumatic event.

Think about finding yourself in a serious car accident. A red SUV ran you over, and you were badly injured. You didn't reflect over the fact that you collided with a red car. After a while, you noticed that you are not comfortable in busy traffic anymore. One explanation can be that, every time you pass by a red car, an SUV, or a red SUV, your unconscious mind recognizes this as a traumatic situation and automatically begins to produce an inner chemical state that makes you feel as if you were back in that traumatic situation. When these types of situations occur, the body controls the brain. The servant has again become the master.

Because the brain always works by repetition and association, a trauma is not required in order for the body to begin to take control over the brain.[88]

Many believe that they think and feel in the present, but they have a body that lives in the past.

We cannot change ourselves if we live in a predictable future. We will lose the moment here and now, which is so important.

You destroy the quantum field if you try to predict a desired event.

A desired event should come as a surprise, not as a predicted event. If you can predict the event, it is not something new. You will produce the same familiar outcome. If you try to control the outcome, you are back to deterministic science, where A leads to B, leading to C.

So-called miracles can be described as individuals who decided that they will change both the way they think and feel and how they physically act so that the body is no longer expressed from the past but, rather, is a map to a better future.

In order to achieve this, they must overcome the environment, the body, and time.

A good example of overcoming the environment, the body, and time is when you feel "in the zone." This is a very common expression in sports. You feel invincible, recover better, handle training better, and sleep better. You have made yourself into a protein-producing machine made for success.

Survival versus creation

In an evolutionary perspective, the development of the prefrontal cortex is a newer development of the human brain, which separates us from animals. We use this part of the brain when we think a specific thought. We know from previous chapters what our thoughts are able to do.

I have previously talked about our defense system. When it concerns the human stress response system, it doesn't always work to our advantage. I will now give an example of how this works seen through the lenses of quantum mechanics.

In both humans and animals, the stress response is turned on automatically when we find ourselves unbalanced. This happens if we are late for an appointment, meet a neighbor who we are having an ongoing argument with, or when the fire alarm goes off. To compare this to the animal world, this happens when a competitor challenges you to fight or a grazing gazelle suddenly catches the eye of a lion running full speed just a few meters away.

The difference is that, in animals, this response will automatically cease when the danger has passed. Among humans, we have a tendency to turn short-term stress into long-term stress by thinking back to the situation that made us produce the stress response in the first place.

Unlike animals, we have the ability to turn on our defense system by just a thought.

Similar to animals, the human body is not made to be in defense mode over a long time. Think back about the gazelle eating grass. The parasympathetic nervous system is active and ensures digestion, growth, and maintenance. As soon as it spots a lion trying to eat it, the gazelle will turn all of the activity pertaining to growth and development and redirect that energy toward the defense system in order for it to work as effectively as possible. The only thing that is important for the gazelle now is to outrun the lion. It is fascinating to see that, within a few minutes after the gazelle has outrun the lion, it will go back to grazing again. It is back to growth and maintenance. If the gazelle behaved as a human, it would probably think back on the situation months after it happened. This stress response would slowly but surely lead to disease and an early death.

Three things are important for a gazelle when a lion attacks. It must attempt to survive (ensure that the body is intact), attempt to run away from the threatening surroundings, and do this as quickly as possible. Do you recognize the three factors—the surroundings, the body, and time?

When these factors are not well addressed, it leads us to be more matter and less energy. Living in defense mode causes us to focus our energy on .00001 percent of reality, instead of the 99.99999 percent, which is energy.

When we consume energy from our surroundings, less will be left over to use on the inner processes, which ensure homeostasis. You get sick more easily, whether it is a cold, cardiovascular disease, or cancer.

Since our senses are based on previous experiences, the use of the senses to define our reality leads to the senses deciding our reality. This is like living based on principles from Newton, where you attempt to control the outcome. You live in order to survive. Is that the kind of life you prefer? One reason it is so common to live by our senses is because our senses operate by time, place, and surroundings. This defines who we are. We become self-centered. In a stressful situation, it would be smart to be self-centered in order to survive. Under chronic stress, both the brain and the body will be unbalanced when our survival mechanisms are prioritized over growth and development. Positive feelings lead you to become unselfish, whereas negative feelings make you self-centered.

We have seen that thoughts can make us sick. The good thing is that thoughts can also make us well. In order to create your own future, you must let your surroundings, body, and time be more like waves and less like particles so that they cannot invade your conscious mind. You must live as if you are nobody. When you're in this state, you will completely forget to be yourself. Meditation is an example of this state.

The frontal lobe of the prefrontal cortex is evolutionarily the newest part of our brain and separates us the most from other living organisms. The frontal lobe controls our attention, presence, consciousness, concentration, and observation. This area is the most adaptable area of the brain and has the function of creating new synapses and changes.

In order to change ourselves, we have to change the frontal lobe. If we are not satisfied with how we function, we must change our way of thinking, feeling, and behaving. Over time, your conscious mind will stop the unconscious mind from activating the undesired networks that represent the person you were before. You stop signaling to the genes in the same way.

You cannot create a new personal reality with the same personality.

When we have erased the old program of who we were before, the next task is to create a new program. In order to do this, it is smart to ask open, curious questions, which enables you to look at your opportunities. If your new thoughts are more real than everything else, you will be on your way to creating your own future.

When you stand in front of the mirror, one day you can see a nice well-trained person, while another day a reflection can show your wrinkles, pimples, and blemishes at the same time. You have certainly not changed so much overnight. Which reflection is correct?

We have now established a viewpoint that we can actively influence our everyday life. Why is it so that many focus on what they don't want instead of what they want?

It seems that it is human nature to wait for change until something is so bad that we can't stand it any longer. This applies to both individuals and society in general. First, when we experience a crisis, an accident, a near-death experience, disease, or tragedy, we begin to evaluate how we live. Why does it have to be a "worst-case scenario" for us to begin to make a change?

It is much easier to avoid putting on weight, rather than getting rid of excess weight. It is easier to avoid depression, rather than finding your way out of depression.

If you are waiting for science to give you permission to do something unusual or something that is not confirmed through scientific studies, then you are in the practice of turning science into a new religion.

What we know today can be wrong tomorrow. What if we are wrong? What if you are lying on your deathbed and realize that you have been wrong your entire life?

Because Western medicine looks at the body as a machine, it is preoccupied with taking control and dominating the body from the outside. Regarding cancer, Western medicine invokes artillery against cancer using chemotherapy and radiotherapy, which without a doubt bring many innocents into the battle. Eastern medicine looks at this in a different way. The body is viewed more holistically. Instead of attacking cancer with the thought of killing it, Eastern medicine attempts to reestablish homeostasis/balance in the body. When the body's inner chemical composition is in harmony, it will be better capable to handle the stress that the body is exposed to.

Back to Claude Bernard—"Illnesses hover constantly above us, their seeds blown by the wind, but they do not set in the terrain unless the terrain is ready to receive them."

There is no doubt that Western medicine has saved many cancer patients from dying of cancer, but we must always remember that a symptom is never the reason but, rather, a consequence of the reason. Maybe it is about time to let our polarized world melt together so that we can take advantage of the best of both worlds.

In a stressful life where the body operates in defense mode during the most of the day, it will be more natural to protect your own decisions and opinions. This leads to polarization and does not just apply to how we look at health, but can also be applicable to religion or politics.

The less we need to protect ourselves from each other, the more energy we can use for growth, development, happiness, and harmony.

What if we are wrong?

We base our lives around stories that have been retold for thousands of years. The stronger we believe in these stories, the more time we spend living by them, and the more we do in order to redistribute them in order to keep them alive. What if these stories are wrong? In an interview with the Dalai Lama, where he was asked what he would have done if he knew that science could prove that parts of Buddhism were incorrect, he responded, "Change Buddhism." You should be open and brave in order to recognize that you have been wrong. You are even braver for making changes in your life that respond to the new knowledge.

A good example is the gene hypothesis, including the human genome project, which has been shown to be incorrect. Most of today's medical practices continue to build upon the hypothesis that it is genes that decide the outcome and that genes are inherited through generations and are rigidly defined without the possibility of change. I have read a study that claims that it takes seventeen years on average until a fact is established and put into practice. Examples from my practice are the medical profession's usage of antibiotics for ear infections among children and the general use of NSAIDs and cortisone steroids (anti-inflammatory drugs). Despite the changing guidelines of the use of these medications, they continue to be poured out as if they were candy. Almekinder already wrote in 1999, "In the absence of advantageous results of simple pain relievers as well the placebo, and the large amount of potential side effects, it is difficult to justify any role of NSAIDs."[89] In an article published in *Aspetar Sports Medicine Journal* in 2013, we can read, "With the potential complications, the familiar, negative influences of muscle regeneration and the natural self-regulation of muscular damage, neither scientific evidence nor WADA Anti Doping Code support anyone's usage of cortisone steroids when it applies to muscle injuries."[90]

Albert Einstein has defined insanity as "doing the same thing over and over again and expecting different results." Many people live in what I call the "comfort zone." Ironically enough, this does not have to be very comfortable. In this setting, comfortable means familiar. We tend to be drawn back to what is familiar. Although we know that something is wrong or that the outcome of our actions probably does not lead to what we hope for, we keep doing the same things over and over again. The servant has become the boss—remember?

3

Science

I finished my preface by giving two simple steps to achieve well-being:

1. You have to find out what is good for you and what is bad for you.
2. You have to do what is good for you and avoid what is bad for you.

Then I gave you two reasons why so many fail to achieve well-being. One of the reasons is that you have to have the right information and many don't.

Much of the information today about what is right and what is wrong comes from science. What if the science we bring forward and base our recommendations on is wrong? Can we trust science? Let's take a closer look.

Has science become religion?

Back in time, those who did not follow the church's point of view were thrown into prison or punished. During the renaissance, people were supposed to have a more open mind regarding knowledge. "Doubt everything" and "I think, therefore I am" are familiar sayings from Descartes.

Over time, science has become synonymous with truth—exactly the same way faith was the truth before the renaissance. It is sensational to see that those who hold science as the absolute truth today are using the same actions the church used in earlier times—prison, fines, and so forth.

Today, we still see examples where people are punished for not following certain scientific treatment methods. In some countries, your child will be refused entrance to public kindergarten or school if he or she is not vaccinated. People are punished if they refrain from using chemotherapy and radiotherapy in treatment of cancer or for giving birth the natural way as opposed to having a recommended Caesarean section. Many of the strongest recommendations exist despite extremely poor documentation.

Is materialistic science making us blind and turning us into a strong faith on the same level that religion has its strong faith? It is interesting to notice that Crick's gene hypothesis is called dogma. By definition, dogma represents a faith-based on religious conviction, not scientific facts!

Before I venture further into what today's science is becoming, I want to point out that I support good research, and I think research is important for future development. Simultaneously, I believe that philosophy-based and knowledge-based practice should go hand in hand and not polarize each other the way they often do today.

Science *must* be based on a philosophy; if not, questions would never have been raised.

The major reason I find it challenging to trust research today is that some of the research is based on a mechanistic, deterministic, and reductionist science. If you ask poor questions, you will most likely get poor answers. In my opinion, there is too much research relying on measurable quantities. Energy and quality are left out. After all, we are living creatures, not mechanistic robots.

My goal is to get you as the reader to make up your own mind. Do not blindly trust what the so-called experts are telling you. Try to look a little behind the recommendations. Is there an economic or political agenda? What sounds reasonable to you and what is in line with your basic philosophy?

When GPs are subscribing medicine or surgery, I believe they do this in the best interest of their patients, because they have been taught to do so—just the same way I choose my recommendations. At times, I do not agree on the medical profession's basic premises.

In the preface, I wrote about how my parents did not question any of the national recommendations but, rather, followed them conscientiously. I don't blame my parents. They did what they were told to do. I blame the system. I think my parents were given some unfortunate recommendations.

It is the same thing with research based on outdated science. I do not think researchers deliberately try to fool you. It is just that sometimes I do not agree on their basic premises.

I will not claim that my point of view and arguments in this book are all correct. It is a big possibility that I am wrong in some aspects, and if I, in retrospect, see that I was wrong, I will change my recommendations. In my twenty years as a practitioner, I have changed my recommendations several times based on newly adapted knowledge. In the span of more than forty years, I have changed my lifestyle several times, and I will most certainly do it again.

I have chosen to refer to a range of studies when I pose arguments for or against something. I am not a researcher. I run a practice where I attempt to help people improve their quality of life. I have no guarantee that the studies that I refer to supporting my points of view are any better than the studies I criticize, which don't support my points of view. The studies that I refer to are found in so-called scientific journals with given criteria of what can be included. I ask you as a reader to be equally critical of those studies I refer to that support my point of view as you are of the studies I criticize. At the end, you will have to add up and figure out what goes with your basic premises.

As a holistic practitioner, it can be frustrating to explain a three-dimensional phenomenon with a two-dimensional tool set. When I speak about tools, I am speaking of so-called evidence-based knowledge.

Some of the evidence-based knowledge is built on outdated scientific theories, which are reductionist, materialistic, and deterministic. It is devoid of nuances and personal evaluations. Context is ignored.

Science will most likely describe a wooden plank based on concrete measurements such as length and width. A carpenter would describe the same piece of wood with the words "deformed," "discolored," "rotten," or "full of twigs." Would you build a house with correct dimensions but poor quality materials? Simultaneously, would you remove the opportunity to evaluate if it is more purposeful to use nails, screws, hammer, a nail gun, a screwdriver, or a power drill from the carpenter?

Is today's science characterizing how we live? Are we being led into a context-free world? These are questions that I reflect upon when I see kids using a drawing program on their iPads. It seems clean and pretty, with sharp, clear colors and without the possibility to draw on the outside. However, what happens to the nuances and all of the sensory impressions? A crayon smells different from a marker. A larger crayon requires a different grip than a thin crayon. A hard pressure applied with the crayon creates a stronger color than does a looser pressure. A pointed crayon creates thinner lines than a blunt crayon. By moving the crayon with a larger motion, we are able to cover a larger area, but it is easier to get color outside of the drawing sheet. With smaller motions, it is easier to be more precise, but it will take more time, and on and on.

In the context of my practice, I also see examples of how we are being led into a context-free world devoid of nuances and personal assessment. Health is, like I mentioned, considered "big business" and a market that the insurance industry has put its eyes upon. Honestly, I do not believe this is because the insurance business cares one bit about your health, but because the industry sees it as an economic profit. Some of the insurance companies in Norway have started their own network. In order to be a part of this network, treatments must undergo a set of guidelines from the insurance companies at the prices the insurance companies require. When a patient needs treatment, an external person who has never met the patient (sometimes located in another country, if the company has outsourced this service) decides the number of consultations needed, the duration of the treatment, and what should be done. The patient is probably assessed based on tables and statistics, which have been compiled through so-called scientific studies. Where are the nuances and personal assessments? This is definitively not best for the patients. I strongly distance myself from such networks.

The medical profession has mentioned evidence-based medicine as a new paradigm.[91] It is claimed that this is a system that ensures that professionals use methods that are scientifically documented to achieve a desired effect.

Science over the last four hundred years has become synonymous with truth, and we can, in other words, operate a quality assured practice based on truths. Maybe it is not so strange that society has pushed the limits of what medicine can achieve to the brink.

But wait, when something is too good to be true, it is often so!

The background of evidence-based practice

The British doctor Archibald Leman Cochrane believed in the 1970s that the medical practice was characterized by traditions and subjective opinions from self-proclaimed experts. He believed that experience-based knowledge leads to committing the same mistake repeatedly. He highlighted more knowledge from research-based studies.[92] Cochrane wanted to develop a system that ensured effects based on statistical trials that revealed methods that either were harmful or had no effect.

After several studies, there was a problem for the practicing doctor because a lot of time was required to know about all these studies. The doctors were not used to this, and it led to a gap between the scientific community and the medical profession.

In order to close this gap, meta-analyses were developed. This is an analysis of results from previous empirical examinations of a phenomenon. These analyses were presented in systematic reviews. It was now possible to summarize conclusions from many sources and manageable to keep updated for those who practiced.

In 1992, *JAMA: The Journal of the American Medical Association* published a manifesto that formulized a new approach to how one should practice medicine. The manifesto was compiled by the Department of Clinical Epidemiology and Biostatistics, McMaster University, Canada.

Evidence-based practice has spread to the entire world and is today coordinated in the Cochrane and Campbell Collaborations. The Nordic Cochrane Center started up back in 1993. In my country, Norway, the Norwegian Knowledge Centre for Health Services was established in 2004.

Characterized by Cochrane's background as an epidemiologist and specialist in biostatistical methods, RCT (randomized control trial) is considered the gold standard within evidence-based medicine. Randomized means that participants of a study have been arbitrarily selected and divided into groups. The control occurs from members of the control group, who receive stimulus that is not real (placebo). This attempts to see whether the effect being measured is the result of the intervention or the placebo effect. RCT's are often double-blinded, meaning neither the participants nor the research conductors themselves know whether the participants belong to the intervention group or the control group.

Evidence-based practice looks at treatment effect, from which scientific methods are used. The strength of the scientific documentation is ranked based on the method, which has created the basis for assessment.

A classic medical hierarchy is divided into five categories. In the bottom category is expert opinion. In category four, there are case studies and weak cohort studies. A case study follows a case or entity in order to see the effect of an intervention. A cohort study follows a group of people over a period of time. In category three, there are single case-controlled studies and systematic reviews over case-control studies. Case-control studies are an analytic model where people with a disease or symptom are compared with healthy people, with the thought of revealing differences regarding the prior influence of possible pathogenic factors. Systematic reviews are obtained from literature studies. On level two, there are single cohort studies, RCTs, and systematic reviews of cohort studies. All the way at the top, we have systematic reviews of RCTs and single RCTs of good quality. It is amazing that qualitative studies and observations are not even assessed in this system.

Let us take a peek behind the scenes.

Evidence-based practice proves to establish a cause-and-effect relationship. We recognize this from Descartes and Newton's determinism. Determinism tries to reveal a linear context, where A leads to B, leading to C. We can probably trace the development of evidence-based knowledge back to this time. A way to see this is by looking at evidence-based knowledge as an attempt to put theories of the 1700s in a system. I have previously pointed out the weaknesses of deterministic science when describing human phenomenon. A common misunderstanding is that the first event causes the second event just because the first event occurred before the next.

It is important to separate compliance (correlation) and cause. There is a difference between being linked to a disease and causing disease. Think about the relationship of a hammer and a carpenter. Most people will associate a hammer with the carpenter, but it is not the hammer itself that conducts the carpentry. It is the person that controls the hammer. The carpenter controls the outcome. We can use a car as another example. A car holds all of the mechanical parts that allow it to drive, but it does not drive anywhere without a driver present, giving the car instructions of what to do. If we use the mechanistic and reductionist approach that conventional medicine often practices, accidents will only occur because of mechanical dysfunctions of the car. The driver will not be considered as causing the accident.

I have a dog. When my dog is happy, it wags its tail. The wagging is an effect of my dog being happy. This can be due to many causes, such as going for a walk, receiving a treat, or becoming excited by cuddles. I cannot make my dog happy by taking its tail and wagging it!

What if I portray this in a different way? Your mood is influenced by your sensory perception of your environment. Mood is an effect of your sensory perception. If you go to your doctor and say that you feel down and depressed and you are offered an antidepressant drug, wouldn't this be strikingly similar to the owner attempting to make his or her dog happy by wagging its tail?

It is difficult to quantify quality and produce statistics out of qualities. As a result, we also see that qualitative studies are not even being assessed in the evidence-based hierarchy.

I believe that the embracement of evidence-based knowledge today is a clear indication that materialism, reductionism, and determinism still stay strong in today's society.

Albert Einstein has said, "The significant problems we face today cannot be solved at the same level of thinking we were at when we created them."

The biggest critique of the evidence movement is that it gives extremely little consideration to context. Neither the environment nor the mind is taken into consideration.

"If we are serious about coming to know something, then our research methods will have to be adapted to the nature of the phenomenon that we are trying to understand ... One may need to draw on the totality of one's experience, and not just on that subset that consists of observations made through the process of traditional scientific discovery."[93]

A vase has its own characteristics because it has the form of a vase. If you break this vase into a thousand pieces, it will have the exact same constituents, but the characteristics will be completely different. Similarly, with humans, you cannot expect to understand humans by picking them apart and studying their parts, without looking at them in their correct context.

You can see with your eyes, but what does it mean if you do not have a brain to interpret the sensory information?

Body and mind cannot be separated. We are a part of a whole. The whole is bigger than its parts. We have previously seen that the placebo effect absolutely plays its part. We have also seen that, essentially, your brain's interpretation decides which response the body reacts with, independent of whether the cause is due to physical, mental, or chemical stimulus. Since the placebo effect is a part of a desired effect, I see big weaknesses with the consideration of RCTs as a gold standard for revealing scientific human facts.

I have previously used a computer analogy to explain how the brain works. This is only a limited explanation. An essential difference is that your brain has emotions, but the computer doesn't. You can tell me your favorite color and if you like carrots or asparagus more. The computer will not be able to give you an answer. Feelings and emotions are not quantifiable. When we do research on humans, when can we exclude emotions? If RCTs are performed based on reductionist, materialistic, and deterministic knowledge, what kind of answers will they give us?

The fact that evidence-based knowledge does not take context into consideration is not something the evidence movement is trying to hide.

The Norwegian Knowledge Center for Health Services writes in its strategy plan for 2005, "The Knowledge Center's role will mostly be connected to evaluating and measuring and not to understand more basic mechanisms or construe experiences and contexts." For me this appears as the reductionist, materialistic, and deterministic philosophy that I mentioned earlier.

This is also congruent with the manifesto that was published by *JAMA* in 1992, which states:

> Evidence-based medicine emphasizes less on intuition, unsystematic clinical experience and pathophysiological rationale as a satisfactory basis for grasping clinical decisions…
>
> In the shortage of systematic observations, one must be careful with the interpretation of information obtained by clinical experience and intuition, because it can sometimes be misleading…
>
> The new paradigm will cherish the authority much lower than the old.

In other words, it is important to exclude everything that makes us able to construe anything.

Which criteria will we have for facts?

I have previously talked about how our inner reality is created by our sensory perception from our senses, which again is based on previous experiences, memory, and expectations. Here is an example.

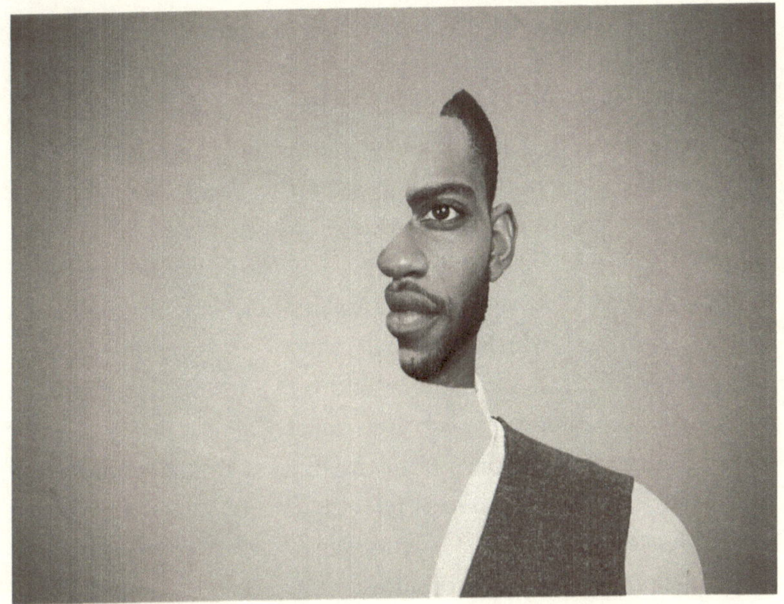

Figure 3.1. Do you see the man from the side or the front?

If you show me a picture of a grouse, I will automatically think about recreation, since I love to be in the mountains and hunt the grouse. If you show the same picture to a chef, it is likely the chef will think about food. If you show the picture to an ornithologist, the ornithologist will most likely think about something like a bird in the poultry family.

A sensory impression is always subjective.

Another characteristic of our brain is that it will fill in the information it lacks based on previous experience. A good example is our ability to read words where the letters are helter-skelter, as long as the first and last letter is correct:

Let us check it out. It deos not mttaer in whcih odrer the leertts are, as lnog as the fsirt and the lsat lettres are cecroret. You can try to make your own stneneecs.

Can you think about how this can influence research based on observation?

Evidence is based on observation. All observation is subjective, based on what is being observed. To establish a cause-effect relationship, there must be a subjective imagination of the proposed hypothesis present; if not, there would be no study. Since study design can be chosen, then it is not objective. Nothing is objective when it concerns issues that someone has an interest in or cares about. In opposition to a computer, humans have emotions. Humans look for answers that confirm their assumptions and overlook more or less known facts, which can dispute them. The more time, energy, and personal interest there are behind our assumptions, the more stubbornly we will look for confirmation.

In addition to the precise measurements, it is also important that what is being measured is relevant. There does not exist any guidelines for this when RCT is applicable. Personal observation, personal opinions, and expert opinions must then be trusted. If you remember from the evidence hierarchy, you will find these factors completely at the bottom of the hierarchy.

Isn't it ironic that a paradigm that has the purpose of excluding subjective interpretation is based on exactly the same?

Isn't it also ironic that there does not exist any evidence that evidence-based practice is more effective than another form of practice?

In evidence-based medicine, the truth becomes defined based on methods, not the assessment of the contents.

Do you remember the previous example with the married couple and their friend discussing dieting? When the man said that his cholesterol had reduced from 8 to 4 by changing to a low carbohydrate diet and all of his adverse reactions from the statins were gone after he stopped taking the drugs, the overweight woman, who even had difficulties walking, strongly disagreed because of the lack of evidence. The man was humble enough to say that he was not sure about the evidence. My question is, what type of evidence would have been good enough for the woman to find it interesting enough to change her dietary intake? The best evidence sat right in front of her.

A ten-year-old boy, along with his father, came to see me at my clinic. The father said that his son had never had a dry night. Every night in the past ten years, he'd wet his bed. In addition to being physically and mentally tiring for the parents to change the boy's clothes and sheets every night, the boy himself was beginning to feel embarrassed. He refused to spend the night at his friend's place. The times when he eventually did, he snuck away to put on a diaper without anyone noticing, before he went to bed.

At this age children begin spending the night outside the home for school and leisure activities. Everyone was concerned. They heard that chiropractic could help, so they paid me a visit. I will not go into the examination findings and treatment plan, but after only two treatments, the boy stopped wetting his bed. A control appointment was booked after two weeks in order to see if the effect lasted. The father canceled this appointment the day before and, on the verge of tears, told me they didn't need the appointment because the boy had not had one single accident after the last treatment. We agreed that they could call me if the problem showed up again. I have not heard anything from them since, but they have certainly referred many other children with the same problem to see me.

Supporters of evidence-based practice will scream for evidence and probably call the effect pure luck or placebo. They should ask the boy, his mother, or his father what type of evidence they need to see?

A five-year-old boy consulted me, together with his father, at the clinic. His right eye didn't work like the left. He had bad stereopsis. He had used a patch over his eye for more than two years without any benefit at all. After several controls, both at his optician's and his doctor's with discouraging results and a continued recommendation of the usage of the patch, the parents began to doubt that this would have an effect. They admitted that they had not been so great at using the patch recently when motivation began to die out. They decided to try an alternative approach, and since I had already helped the mother, father, and older sister with different health-related problems, they decided to take the one and a half-hour car trip to see me. Without going into details of the examination, findings, or adjustments, it was extremely pleasing to hear that the eye test with the eye doctor one week after the boy was adjusted finally showed huge progress.

I do not have good evidence that satisfies the evidence-based movement for either of these two cases. I cannot support my treatment with double-blinded RCTs that show that everyone who has had a vision defect or wets the bed will become better by the particular adjustments I performed on these two boys.

Thus, I do not have any problems with giving a neurological explanation of what I think led to the desired effect. The explanation is based on acquired knowledge from years of health-related studies; tens of thousands of patient consultations; empirical evidence from colleagues; and, finally yet importantly, a burning desires to help my patients.

This is unfortunately not considered proof within evidence-based practice. I often hear these types of results are based on coincidence, patients being tricked or being dumb, or patients who throw away money on something that is not scientifically proven.

It could be considered a coincidence when the ten-year-old boy suddenly had his first dry night after the adjustment. The same could be said for the five-year-old boy who used a patch over his eye for more than two years without any progress, when he suddenly experienced a huge progress on a vision test one week after being adjusted. I see similar examples in my clinic on a regular basis. You can decide yourself what you believe is more probable—effect from the treatment or pure luck.

Daily, I experience results in the clinic that I cannot explain based on evidence-based practice. Sometimes I also experience results that I cannot explain at all. Regardless, I cannot deny the results. My job is to try to understand the mechanisms behind these different results.

What do you think the ten-year-old, the five-year-old, or their parents would consider good enough evidence? What if I said that we were no longer allowed use treatments that aren't proven through evidence-based guidelines? Unfortunately, that is not far away from where we are today.

What consequences could exclusion have?

When there is a selection of relevant information, other information might be excluded. In another context, or with new knowledge, the information excluded can be equally important or more important than the information chosen. If we stop posing critical questions to given truths, science will be dogmatic.

All new theories are developed because someone was critical of existing truths. If we lived by one truth, further development would end. Albert Einstein said, "Imagination is even more important than knowledge. For while knowledge defines all we currently know and understand, imagination points to all we might yet discover and create."

Evidence-based medicine often lacks evidence in its foundation, and there is no evidence that shows that evidence-based medicine has a better effect than anything else. In addition to appearing as superhuman, infallible and immortal, it emerges as a considerable authority. Evidence-based medicine comes forward as a paradigm that is based on *faith* and *authority*.

It is interesting that the definition of dogma is "a term used when a *faith* or doctrine as in many types of belief systems and organizations become praised as *authoritative*, or as absolute truth ... Many non-religious perceptions often become referred to as dogma, for example within philosophy, science, politics and in society in general. The term alludes to when humans hold on tightly to their own perception in a one-sided and non-reflective way. Dogma is often seen as non-existent in scientific and philosophical contexts, but it can occur among these groups as well" (*Wikipedia*).

It is not just the structure of evidence-based medicine that is dogmatic. The science that it is based on is also dogmatic. Take, for example, the gene hypothesis, which was set forth by Watson and Crick. This hypothesis, which was meant to confirm and map out genes based on the gene hypothesis, was proven to be wrong through the Human Genome Project in 2001.

It is a problem for the critics of the evidence movement that evidence-based practice identifies itself with science. Signs of similarity are often created between "evidence-based" and "scientific-based," simultaneously as "science" is understood as a synonym of "knowledge." This means that critics appear to be unintelligent or unappreciative of knowledge. Paradoxically, practicing clinicians who do not blindly embrace evidence-based medicine are often accused of giving treatments based on faith rather than facts, using spiritual treatment, or simply engaging in trickery.

Albert Einstein once said, "Great spirits have often encountered violent opposition from mediocre minds."

I remember back to the time where I was about to choose where I would study physiotherapy. One college claimed that its method of instruction was knowledge-based. That sounded great, but what did the other institutions base their education on? I wondered.

What if I claim that this knowledge is based on outdated science, a science assumed to be the truth?

RCT as the gold standard

The gold standard for research today is called a double-blinded randomized controlled trial (RCT).

The method has the purpose of answering whether a measure has an effect to a significant degree. This is measured exclusively by evaluating procedures and methods. The focus is on *how* we know something, not *what* we know. In order to draw a conclusion from an RCT, it is also irrelevant why something has an effect as long as it has one. It is enough to know that it works—not different from what people in the old days called magic!

In order to illustrate how evidence-based medicine can be seen in a sarcastic way, a study was published in *The BJM* (*British Medical Journal*) in 2003, with the title "Parachute Use to Prevent Death and Major Trauma Related to Gravitational Challenge: Systematic Review of Randomized Controlled Trials."[94]

Result: They were not able to find any RCTs of parachute intervention.

> Conclusion: As with many interventions intended to prevent ill health, the effectiveness of parachutes has not been subjected to rigorous evaluation by using randomized controlled trials. Advocates of evidence-based medicine have criticized the adoption of interventions evaluated by using only observational data. We think that everyone might benefit if the most radical protagonists of evidence-based medicine organized and participated in a double blind, randomized, placebo-controlled, crossover trial of the parachute.

When we look at the support around evidence-based medicine, there is no doubt that it is a powerful tool. There is also no doubt that it is a good tool, when it is used correctly and the context is unimportant or context is actually being taken into consideration. However, when is the context really unimportant when it has something to do with human phenomena? RCT based on reductionist, mechanistic, and deterministic knowledge becomes an extremely limited tool, especially due to alternative—and complementary—medical therapy that especially emphasizes context and individually customized treatment.

Ask yourself this question: If you had a serious disorder, would you like to be treated by a naive clinician without experience, who exclusively uses studies and statistics for support, or a clinician who has treated hundreds or thousands of similar cases?

Let us look closer at hypertension as an example. RCT will be a good choice of method if the purpose is to reveal whether a blood pressure-lowering medicine has an effect or not. This is independent of what is causing the high blood pressure or how the medicine will eventually reduce the blood pressure. The study can be done as a double-blind, where neither the investigator nor the test subject knows whether the subject has received medicine or placebo. If there are enough test subjects, this could lead to a statistical significance, with conclusions regarding whether the blood pressure medicine reduces blood pressure. In order to emphasize my point, let me say this: Evidence-based medicine has been a success, and it doesn't matter whether a patient with medically regulated blood pressure dies early, as long as the patient does not die with high blood pressure.

If a patient with hypertension consults a holistic therapist, this therapist will probably have a completely different approach. I can only speak for myself as a practicing chiropractor and physiotherapist—neither bad luck nor bad genes cause hypertension. Rather, hypertension is almost always the result of inappropriate lifestyle, and it is the body's innate defense mechanism in order to reestablish homeostasis in the body. I do not think primarily about what I will do to lower a patient's blood pressure. I look more closely at what is the cause of the hypertension. If this is a lifestyle problem, then there is nothing wrong with the body, and it is doing exactly what it is made to do. What do you think will happen to your blood pressure if you are exercising, holding a lecture in front of two hundred people, or running to catch the bus? We are talking about supply and demand. The body prioritizes the most important tasks first. Giving blood pressure-lowering medicine to someone with hypertension due to bad lifestyle choices is like covering a warning sign in your car, while pretending that nothing is wrong and continuing to drive.

It can be harmful to have a consistently high blood pressure, I agree. As a holistic chiropractor I ask myself *why* the blood pressure is consistently high and how can I contribute with treatment or information to lowering the blood pressure on the premises of the body? For one person, a subluxation of the neck can be the cause. For another person, it can be inactivity. A third might be overweight. A fourth might be overtraining. A fifth might have social stress; a sixth, financial stress; and a seventh, trauma. For an eighth, the culprit might be increased salt intake; for a ninth, poor nutrition; for a tenth, a pain condition; and on and on.[95] The list is almost infinite, and it is often not just one cause but several simultaneously. How can we create RCTs that support customized holistic treatment for our patients?

Think of an experiment where you have a certain amount of dying plants; as a researcher, you want to test out a hypothesis about whether or not water is good for the plants. Without knowing what you are giving, you give water to half of the plants and "fake water" to the other half (blinded study). Result: None of the plants become better. The conclusion from an allopathic viewpoint is that water is not good for plants.

If you put on the holistic hat, you know of course that plants need more than just water.

If we take the experiment a little further, you think that you now want to test out a hypothesis about whether water *and* sun is good for plants. You divide the plants into four groups—of course randomly chosen—and you do not know what you are giving to the plants. Group I receives real water and real sun, group II receives real water and "fake sun," group III receives real sun and "fake water," group VI receives "fake water" and "fake sun." Result: None of the plants become better. All are still dying.

The conclusion from an allopathic viewpoint will be that neither water nor sun is good for plants! You put on the holistic hat again, and you know of course that plants need more than just water and sun.

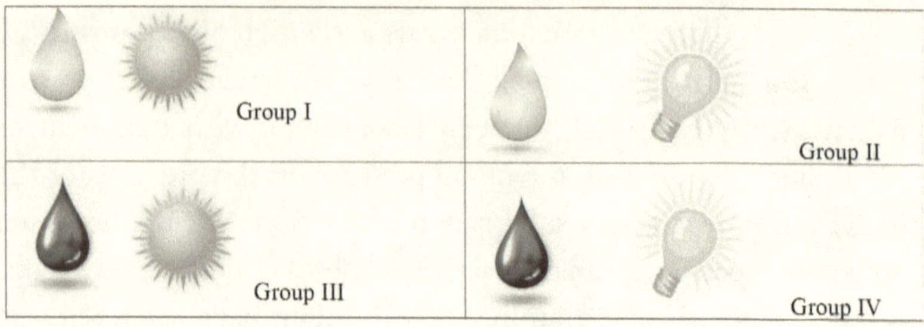

Figure 3.2

We could continue the experimentation by adding plant nutrition, temperature, humidity, and so on. But the point is that it is important what type of questions we ask. If we pose a reductionist question, we receive a limited answer. If the questions are compiled from outdated knowledge, this will give bad conclusions. The question in this particular experiment should be, What brings the plants closer to homeostasis?

What is the definition of "better" in our experiment? From an allopathic view, it will be whether the plants are dying or not. From a holistic view, it will be whether the plants are closer to homeostasis or not. From the holistic point of view, the conclusion will be that all plants that receive "real" stimulus will be closer to homeostasis and, thus, be favorable, although the plant is still dying.

Homeostasis means to be in balance. What if we in our experiment had given too much water or sun? Quantity is also an important factor that we must take into consideration when we assess effect. It is not better to have too much of something than to have too little. Just the right fit will always be just right. When we take into account that humans are considerably more complex than a plant, we can understand, based on the examples above, how difficult it is to handle research concerning humans.

Let us draw a parallel from the dying plant described above and a sore lower back. There can be numerous causes for a sore lower back. Did the pain arise after bending forward, backwards, or sideways or in rotation? Did it start gradually without a particular reason, or is it triggered just by sitting or just by moving? Is the pain acute or has it been there for a while? Is the patient young or old, fit or in bad condition? You surely understand that not all of these possibilities can be treated in the same way.

My patients are living organisms, and they change every day. They will give me the answer. If they change, I must also change my actions in line with their changes. The treatment is tailor-made for every single person and is under constant evaluation and change. It will simply not function if I, as an example, gave all lower back patients four to six treatments where they lay on their right side and I adjusted L5 (bottom lower vertebrae) from the left side each time.

This is unlike allopathic conventional medicine, where high blood pressure, high cholesterol levels, inflammation, or pain respectively will be treated with blood pressure-lowering, cholesterol-lowering, anti-inflammatory, or painkilling medicine, independent of factors such as cause, duration, age, and gender. Since the contrast in causes and characteristics of patients is major, it should be obvious that we cannot treat based on the same criteria.

Often when systematic research reviews do not manage to prove to be statistically significant, it is not because the studies can prove that *whatever treatment is being tested doesn't* have effect. Rather, it may be that *the study* doesn't manage to reveal an effect (nets a false negative result).

There is a current level of misconception from many today that it is being concluded that something does not have an effect when studies cannot prove that they have an effect (false negative). Lacking evidence of an effect is not evidence of lacking effect.[96] Think back to my examples with the ten-year-old bed-wetter or the five-year old with the visual defect. I did not have any scientifically proven evidence to support the outcome, but that is not the same as having evidence that what I did do didn't have the desired effect.

RCT for most alternative and complementarily medical therapies is like choosing the hammer over the whole tool set when a house is being built. To support oneself with Cochrane for evidence for the same therapies becomes like looking for knitting patterns in a motor magazine. You cannot, on the basis of lacking knitting patterns in a motor magazine, conclude that knitting patterns do not exist.

Where ethical considerations come into play, there are challenges. The Helsinki declaration from the World's Doctors Association (1991) says, "The care for test subjects' interests must always be tipped in relation to the interests of science and society." This apparently comes forward in studies where children are involved. There are very little RCTs, concerning children. This applies to both allopathic medicine and alternative and complementary medical therapies.

Many people are skeptical of chiropractic because there does not exist sufficient evidence through RCTs. This also applies to chiropractic for children.

Despite that conventional medicine itself has minimal evidence-behind treatment, medication, advice, or other recommendations, many are critical of chiropractic applied to children on exactly the same basis.

In order to put this into perspective, I will tell you about an event that I was told by a colleague from the United States. My colleague was participating in a debate discussing the treatment of children. He knew that one of the other debaters was a sharp critic of chiropractic in general and especially of chiropractic practice on children. Before the debate, my colleague did some pre-investigations on this critic and found out that he'd recently had a bypass operation on his heart.

As expected this critic "shot from the hip" and accused chiropractic of being based on faith instead of science, saying that it was directly harmful, unethical, trickery, and so on and so forth. My colleague responded that he wanted to be sure that they played with the same applicable rules before they discussed the theme further. He wondered what the critic would recognize as good enough evidence in order for him to accept that chiropractic could have a good effect on children. The critic responded that RCTs were the gold standard and would be needed to prove that chiropractic could have an effect on children. My colleague then followed up by asking if it was true that he'd had a bypass operation of his heart, whereupon the critic confirmed this.

Then, my colleague pointed out that there does not exist any RCTs to support bypass operations up to today's date. He wondered how the critic could choose to be put to sleep in full narcosis and have his chest split open in order to have an operative intervention on the heart, without a single bit of evidence that it would have a positive outcome?

The critic took the bait, became riled up, and fired back about how the heart functioned. Of course it was smart to change a clogged blood vessel, which supplied the heart. Everyone should understand this, and it was unnecessary to have an RCT in order to justify such an operation.

My colleague responded by asking if he agreed that the brain and the nervous system were the main control organs in the body, something the critic was in agreement about. He thus followed up by asking if the critic also agreed that children had a nervous system and whether he considered it important that the nervous system is intact. The critic was silent the rest of the debate.

This example illustrates that we must play by the same rules and the same preconditions. How could this critic blindly rely on background knowledge and experience on such a serious event as a bypass operation and simultaneously promote fearmongering against adjustments of children on the background of missing RCTs? I do not think that my colleague, or myself for that matter, would be in disagreement that a bypass operation is a good solution if one of the heart's veins were clogged. The point is that we cannot prove everything with RCTs. We should give plausible explanation models based on the entirety, not its parts.

From my clinical experience

I wish evidence-based medicine/practice could be illustrated in this way:

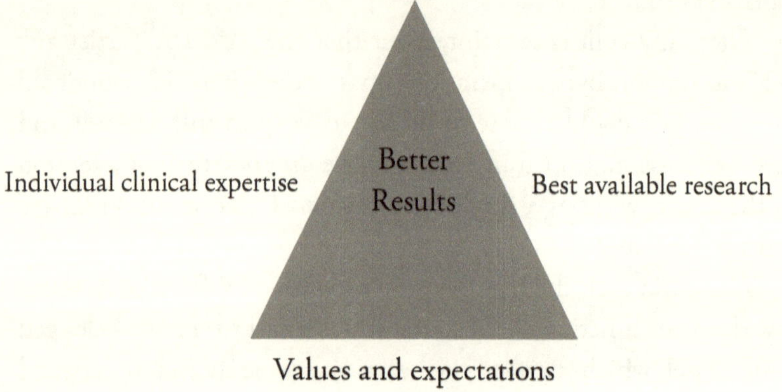

Figure 3.3

Sacket et al. (2000) defines evidence-based medicine as "the integration of the best research evidence with clinical expertise and patient values." This is like music to my ears, but reality is experienced as something completely different.[97]

As a holistic chiropractor and physiotherapist, I help children with ear infections. This treatment is controversial because of lack of evidence. Unfortunately, we do not have scientific evidence in the form of RCTs, but there exist many case studies that are published in scientific journals, which show good results.

I would also like to emphasize that there is no evidence that chiropractic does not work with this group of patients.

Since it is controversial to apply chiropractic to kids with ear infections, I would like to bring up how I will argue to do so, based on what I put in evidence-based practice.

As with all diseases, disorders. or the absence of optimal health, we must remember that the body is complex. We must see humans in their entirety.

There can be many causes of otitis media, but two things are certain—you do not get an ear infection because you are born with too many body parts or by lack of antibiotics!

As a chiropractor, I choose to see patients as human beings, perfectly created but, for one reason or another, not in homeostasis anymore. My job is to find out why they are no longer in homeostasis. This also applies to children with otitis media. The way I see it, there are two reasons why a child gets otitis media.

1.   Bad drainage in the ear
2.   Impaired immune function

The neck, the two upper vertebrae especially, shares nerve innervation, musculature, and structure with the inner ear and sinuses. A dysfunction in this area can lead to impaired drainage to the surrounding structures. This includes not just the ear, but also the throat, nose, and lymphatic system.

There is a hypothesis that children get otitis media because they have more horizontal ear canals than adults. This is also claimed to be the reason children often grow out of otitis media—due to the ear canals becoming more vertically positioned when the cranium grows.

All children have more horizontal ear canals than adults, I agree. If this is the reason for the infections, the question should be, Why doesn't every child suffer from ear infections?

Movement has an important task when it comes to drainage. A dysfunction in the neck will often cause impaired movement, tension in the neck musculature, and possible impaired function of the lymphatic system, which can further lead to reduced drainage. It is often the smallest children who suffer from otitis media. A possible hypothesis could be that the reason children grow out of this problem is that they develop better head control and move around more when they become older.

Structures in the upper part of the spinal cord and in the brain stem are important for the immune system. A dysfunction of the spinal column can lead to impaired immune function. Many believe that the cause of otitis media is bacteria and virus. I do not agree that this is the *cause*. Rather, I believe that this is a consequence of an impaired immune system. I am quite sure that parents reading this, who have had children with otitis media and have several children, have noticed that it is extremely rare that all children have otitis media simultaneously. Why does one child develop otitis media and not the others if the children reside in the same surroundings and bacteria and virus are the cause? The cause being attributed to bacteria comes from the "germ theory," which I have elaborated on earlier in this book.

Today, we have billions of bacteria in our bodies, most of which are good bacteria, which our lives are dependent on. Maybe we receive the most important of them through the birth canal when we are born. To be born by the help of the C-section will not give the baby a boost of the immune system. Furthermore, we develop a good immune system through breast milk. Immune globulins are larger proteins found in breast milk. In order for them to have an effect on children, the child must have a "leaky gut." This makes it possible for these immune globulins to pass through the intestinal wall and reach the bloodstream so that the child develops a good immune system. It requires that the mother is healthy and has these immune globulins. If the child is not breastfed, he or she would most likely receive pasteurized cow's milk or replacements, which the body doesn't manage to utilize in the same way. Since children have "leaky guts", larger unwanted proteins such as casein will go out into the bloodstream with the possibility of influencing the health in a negative way.

Many also claim that otitis media is genetic. This is a hypothesis that was thoroughly torn apart and disproved by the Human genome Project in 2003. There exists absolutely no evidence that we are born with genes that will give us otitis media.

My approach to treating otitis media will be to achieve better drainage and a better immune system. More specifically, this will include adjusting possible dysfunctions in the spine. An adjustment on a child is extremely gentle and does not constitute more pressure than the pressure applied on a closed eye without discomfort. I will give advice about staying away from sugar, milk products, and refined carbohydrates, and I often advise a supplementation of probiotics. If the child is older, I give advice about being physically active. I also use time to defuse these bothers. It is not dangerous if it hurts, you get a fever (until a certain limit), or puss/ liquid comes out of the ear. This is the body's physiology in action, trying to adapt itself to the condition.

If the parents seem interested, I also spend time explaining how the ear functions.

There is no evidence that antibiotics help against otitis media or upper respiratory tract infections in general. Conventional medicine has also established this view. In the *Journal of the Norwegian Medical Association*, it is also stated that it is not recommended to give antibiotics for inflammation of the ear. We also know that antibiotics have a range of side effects, both short-term and long-term, and that excessive use of antibiotics can lead to resistance. I think I have yet to experience a child coming to my clinic with otitis media who has not received antibiotics if he or she has seen a doctor first!

Since chiropractic builds on holistic principles, it is difficult to prove the effect by using reductionist and mechanistic science. On the other hand, there exists a lot of empirical proof among children, parents, and chiropractors that our approach can have good results. Since our approach has few (soreness, tenderness) or no side effects, I see no qualms in justifying my treatment. The way I see it, this is the best available knowledge we have today regarding otitis media.

Children do not need more medicine or surgery in order to become better.

Chiropractic

My view on health care is colored by my education within chiropractic and a chiropractic philosophy. This is not a book about chiropractic, but I want to highlight where chiropractic stands in relation to what I have discussed previously in *I Believe in Life* before *Death!* I would like to point out that this is my view of chiropractic through the way I was taught and my interpretation.

As previously mentioned, chiropractic has a philosophical and scientific foundation, as well as being based on the art of practicing.

A range of books has been written about chiropractic philosophy. I will only offer a small part from the foundation of my profession. "One question was always uppermost in my mind in my search for the cause of disease. I desire to know why one person was ailing and his associate, eating at the same table, working in the same shop, at the same bench, was not. Why? What difference, was there in the two persons that caused one to have pneumonia, catarrh, typhoid or rheumatism, while his partner, similarly situated, escaped? Why?"[98]

We have previously seen how the environment influences our health. Chiropractic realizes that the environment play a significant role in people's health. Proper nutrition, movement, and healthy thoughts are all examples of important external factors within chiropractic philosophy. Chiropractic goes a little bit deeper in the understanding of the term "cause". Why does a forming fungus not spread from one foot to infect the other? How can one have swollen tonsils just on one side? How can one have pneumonia on only one side? Don't both lungs breath in the same air? How does a person get only one infected kidney? Isn't the same blood being circulated throughout the entire body? How can only a part of the body become weak without the entire body becoming weak?

B. J. Palmer, D. D. Palmer's son stated later on, "While other professions are concerned with a changing environment to suit the weakened body, Chiropractic is concerned with strengthening the body to suit the environment."

I will illustrate this concept in figure 3.4.

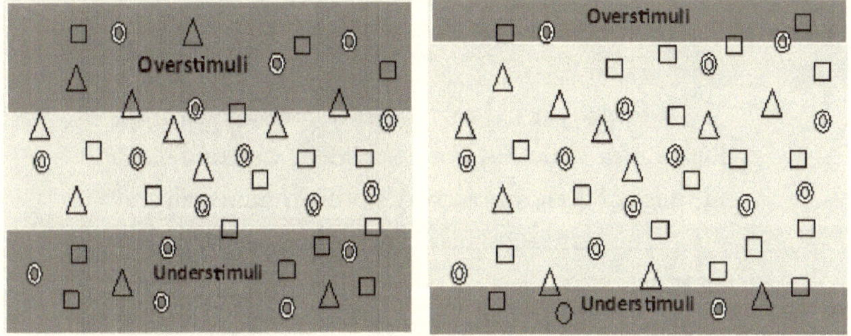

Figure 3.4

The body is dependent on stimulation in order to survive. However, too much is no better than too little. In figure 3.4, the squares indicate physical load, the circles indicate mental load, and the triangles indicate chemical load. The light gray area indicates how much your body is able to adapt. If the dots fall outside of the light gray area and into the dark gray area, we are experiencing a greater change than we can handle. It will bring us away from homeostasis and toward disease and misery.

In the box to the right, we see that the light gray area is narrower. Several of the markers are either in the upper or lower dark gray areas. This means that the adaptability is reduced in relation to the previous box. Previous loads that were within our adaptability range are now found on the outside. The amount of load that was previously good for us has now become the opposite.

I will also illustrate this with an example.

Version 1

A forty-year-old man, who's had the same office job for twenty years, has gotten a lateral epicondylitis. A lateral epicondylitis is popularly known as tennis elbow. He says that this began after he was working with a hammer for an entire weekend.

Version 2:

A forty-year-old man with the same office job for twenty years has gotten a lateral epicondylitis. He has not done any activities other than usual, and his pain started gradually without any particular reason.

In the first instance, I assume that there is a local overload due to the hammering that is the cause of his pain, since the hammering is an unusual activity for the patient. The physical load (squares) is now in the very top in the dark gray area. To help the man, I would focus on relieving measures and try to promote the healing process in the overloaded muscle.

In the second version, I assume that the man's adaptability is slowly but surely becoming poorer and poorer. As a result, it eventually led to an injury. The gray area has become narrower. Load was previously within the adaptability range but now has gradually found itself on the outside. I would now think comprehensively in order to find out the cause of the reduced adaptability. One hypothesis is that the nerves that send signals to the injured muscle group are not optimal. For example, if only three-fourths of the muscle receives signals, the same amount of activity that the muscle previously has handled could now lead to an overload. Another hypothesis is that the patient slowly but surely developed a slouched posture with rounded shoulders resulting in an increased compensatory usage of the musculature in the arm, thus resulting in an overload. The third hypothesis is that something in his office was changed. He could possibly have received a new keyboard, mouse, desk, or chair. He could have changed to another office or something similar—some type of a change from normality. A fourth hypothesis could be that the total amount of stress to the body was too large or recovery was just too little.

Chiropractic is about increasing adaptability, which is represented by the light gray areas in the figures above. Do you remember the studies previously referred to in this book that showed that, as long as a person had a positive sensory reaction to mental stress, then stress was not harmful? On the contrary, the studies showed that stress could have favorable effects. This is absolutely in line with my chiropractic philosophy. As long as the stress or load falls within our tolerance level, it is not destructive. On the other hand, if stress/load is on the outside of our tolerance level, this will lead to disease and misery.

Frederick H. Barge, DC, PhC believed that the cause of disease was the body lacking the ability to adjust itself to its environment.

Sir William Osler once said, "Ask not what kind of illness the patient has, ask what kind of patient has the illness."

"Health is the state of being when the body's physiological homeostatic vitality (tone) is working consistent with the needs of itself and its environment" (Frederick H. Barge, DC, PhC).

Problems arise when the body is unbalanced or no longer in homeostasis. This is due to there being either too much or too little of something. "Something" can be a physical component, such as incorrect load or inactivity. "Something" can be a mental component, such as negative thoughts or financial or relationship problems. "Something" can be a chemical component, such as improper nutrition or toxins.

Three main categories influence us as humans.

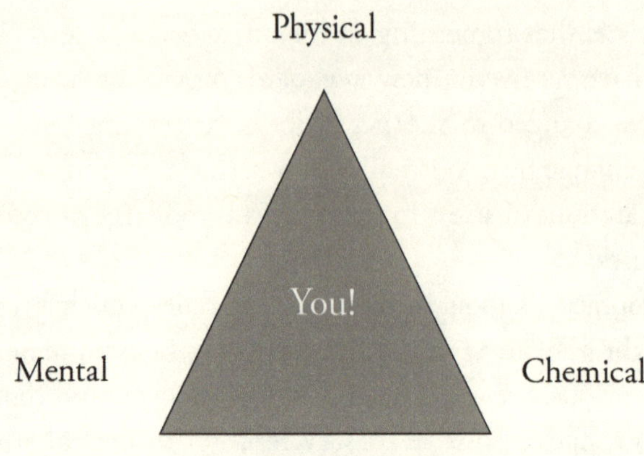

Figure 3.5

These three factors can also be called lifestyle factors. They are the reason unfavorable lifestyle choices lead to bad health. In chiropractic philosophy, this is called "the triune of health."

Favorable environment combined with high adaptability are a good recipe for a long and healthy life.

Innate Intelligence

"The expression of this intelligence through matter is the Chiropractic meaning of life."[99] Chiropractic is founded on what we call "innate intelligence." It means that the body has an innate ability to repair itself or bring itself back to homeostasis. This occurs when a bruise heals or blood pressure adjusts itself in regards to the environment. This expression is named "innate intelligence" and not "innate stupidity" because chiropractic builds its philosophy on the basis that we are created for wellness. "Innate stupidity" would be an appropriate term if we were created for disease and misery.

In this book, I have previously used stress and blood pressure as examples of how the body adjusts itself in order to maintain homeostasis. Another example of this is the regulation of blood sugar. The pancreas must simply work harder to produce insulin if the body is supplied with a lot of sugar. If this happens over a long period of time, the pancreas will become "tired," and the quality of insulin will decrease. The pancreas eventually will not be able to produce sufficient amounts of insulin, which will again lead to a high blood sugar level. As this persists, a person will develop type 2 diabetes. If someone is supplied with external insulin, homeostasis will be recovered, as far as blood sugar is concerned. However, if lifestyle changes are not implemented, cells in the pancreas will die, which creates a dependency on artificial insulin for the rest of ones lives. If the cause of an increased need for insulin production was addressed instead, homeostasis would have been reestablished on the body's own terms, without the dependence on artificially supplied insulin and without side effects. Continued homeostasis would require that one continue with a healthy lifestyle.

"Disease is a lack of coordination between Innate, the source of power, and its expression."[100]

This saying resembles much of what neuroscience shows today. Energy and the brain's function are significant and cannot be left out, as has been the case for centuries.

Chiropractic is furthermore based on the brain being the main controlling center that controls all of the body's functions. The brain sends its signals through an intricate network of nerves between the central nervous system (the brain and the spinal cord) and the rest of the body. This network breaches from the spinal column.

It is not without reason that the skull, which encloses the brain, is hard and protective and that the spinal cord lies well protected inside the spinal column. This implies the importance of taking care of the nervous system. There is also a good reason that the spinal column is made up of 24 free spinal vertebrae. The 24 spinal vertebrae allow us to move our spine, as the central nervous system simultaneously lies well protected inside the spinal column.

Symptoms are the body's natural alarm. Symptoms arise in order to tell us that something in the body is not right. Choosing painkillers as the only treatment for pain relief is the same as taking out a fire alarm's battery whenever the alarm goes off because of the uncomfortable noise. Painkillers will never affect the cause of symptoms! They will only mask them. If the cause of the symptoms persists, you are allowing something harmful in your body to continue by masking the symptoms. Cells are broken down and important functions shut down. The end result could be an early death. This is like letting your house burn down while you pretend that nothing is happening. After a short period, a fire extinguisher is no longer sufficient, and the fire department must be called in if there is even any hope left to save your home.

"Pain is as natural as comfort, the former is a product of disharmony, while the latter is the result of harmony" J. H. Tilden, MD.

The molecular changes that come from a disease are not the cause of the disease; rather, they are the result. The molecular changes confirm the presence of the disease. Symptoms can be the brain's attempt to alert you to the fact that something in the body is not right. Eventually, the brain will not be able to interpret the signals from the body and the environment in a good way.

"It is unfavorable that so few appreciate from what small causes diseases come" Charles H. Mayo, MD.[101]

Statistics from the Institute of Public Health (the Norwegian Prescription Database) show that we used 727,488,704 kroner on prescribed painkillers in 2014 (1600 kroner [200 US dollars] per inhabitant). When we also know that half of us use prescription-free painkillers at least once a week, the amount becomes extremely high. Based on these numbers, there is no doubt that allopathy (treatment of symptoms) continues to stand strong in today's society.[102]

There is an essential difference between chiropractic's fundamental philosophy and conventional medicine's fundamental philosophy:

Medicine: The study of disease and what causes a man to die.

Chiropractic: The study of health and what causes a man to live (C. S. Gonstead, DC).

We need both, but we have to acknowledge the difference.

Healthy choices do not last forever

Most of us have a certain understanding that material things need to be maintained. If you own a car, then you probably take it for servicing occasionally. If you have a house, it will eventually need a paint job. This should be the case with the body as well. Many assume that the body is maintenance free and take little care of their own health. Little action is taken before the pain becomes so massive that it begins to affect one's quality of life and the pain becomes unbearable. As I have previously claimed, symptoms are the body's way of saying that something is not the way it should be. It often begins small. If nothing is done, the symptoms will develop, and the body will probably respond even stronger next time in order for you to understand that something must be done.

When someone asks me for advice regarding what should be done in order to take care of his or her own health, I always reply with the question, What do you like to do? Firstly, they will experience a much better effect from something they enjoy doing as opposed to something they dislike. A study from 2001 showed that bicep strength increased by 13.5 percent after a few weeks by just thinking about contracting the muscle as hard as possible five times a week.[103] A study from 1992 showed that a group who performed finger exercises five times a week for one hour over a four weeks period gained an average increase in finger strength by 30 percent compared to a control group who did not perform any form of training.[104] It is interesting that the group who only thought about performing these exercises five times a week in a four-week period had an average increase in strength by 22 percent. You should absolutely be physically as well as mentally present in order to not waste your time when you work out.

There is also a greater chance that you will continue with the activity if the activity is pleasurable. Your physical condition is perishable and requires that you maintain a certain level of activity. You cannot maintain good health throughout your lifetime by just working out effectively for one or two months. How active do you have to be during your life in order to stay healthy? How many healthy meals do you have to eat in life in order to stay healthy? How much sleep do you need in order to stay healthy? How many good thoughts do you have to think in order to stay healthy? If you are looking for numbers, you are on the wrong track. A healthy lifestyle is required and should be an ongoing process in order to stay healthy.

I feel a little frustrated when I hear people talk about the low-carb diet. Most people connect diets with something that lasts for a short period. I am sure that those who believe that people should eat fewer carbohydrates intend for this to be on a general basis for the rest of one's life, not only during a short period.

It must also be taken into consideration that everyone is different. What works well for some may not work so well for others. We should also remember that life is a dynamic process, and things that were once good for us in the past are not necessarily good for us later in life. Healthy choices should always be adjusted to the person's health status.

For example, many believe that exercising is a good thing regardless of everything. My experience shows that exercise can place someone in a lot more trouble if training is not adapted to the physical level or exercising is performed incorrectly. This clearly shows up in team sports.

Physical condition can simply be divided by strength, endurance, and mobility. When teams of around twenty individuals are always working out in a similar way, there are bound to be some differences. Some individuals need more endurance training, others require strength training, and others need more mobility training. In order to have the best possible effect, good examination methods are required—examinations that evaluate function instead of injury/

disease. As I have pointed out, this is a challenge since classical conventional medicine has a focus on disease and injury, not health and optimal function. Chiropractic is an excellent tool to evaluate function. Athletes are not any different than other people. It should be useful for everyone to obtain one's own health status. This makes it easier to implement ones own measures based on one's goals and conditions.

"The really good physician prevents disease; he cannot cure anything. Because of this knowledge, sickness has become more natural, or more to be expected, than health."[105]

"The maintenance of health should take precedence over the treatment of disease."[106]

Since conventional medicine has a foundation in disease and emergency relief, there are, unfortunately, many who believe that a person is healthy as long as he or she is symptom-free. I have previously mentioned that the first symptom of cardiovascular disease could be death.

We should be thankful for emergency relief. Most of us need emergency relief in the span of our lives. The problem is that emergency relief is related to disease or trauma and has little in common with good health. In order for us to become a healthier population, we need more people to stay healthy. We do not need more people who are being treated for sickness.

Doctor means teacher. As a doctor, one of my primary tasks should be to educate patients about what they can do to contribute to good health and what they should avoid doing in order to avoid becoming sick. This quality is lacking in many doctors today. Education is based on technical skills and an allopathic thought process where patients are fitted into statistics compiled from double-blinded RCTs.

"Most physicians have lost the pearl that was once an intimate part of medicine—humanism. Machinery, efficiency, precision have driven us from the heart warmth, compassion, sympathy and concern for the individual. Medicine is now an icy science. Its charm belongs to another age. The dying man can get little comfort from the mechanical doctor."[107]

A large part of the chiropractic profession emphasizes preventive measures in its practice. A retrospective study of a standardized eighteen-week protocol with a focus on optimal health showed improvements in weight, heart frequency, blood pressure, strength, BMI, and vital capacity. This protocol focused on proper nutrition, supplements, training, and one-on-one counseling, in addition to subluxation-based chiropractic. Chiropractic was not used for symptom relief but because of dysfunctions. In the spinal column, dysfunctions can negatively influence the nervous system and possibly influence both organs and general wellness.[108]

From a mechanical to a neurological explanation model

In 1895, Harvey Lillard had suffered from significant hearing loss for seventeen years. He explained that his deafness arose acutely as he found himself in a crouched position, where he suddenly felt his back give way. During a visit to D. D. Palmer, the founder of chiropractic and who at the time practiced magnetic healing, D. D. Palmer discovered that one vertebra in Lillard's back did not move properly. He adjusted this segment, and Harvey Lillard immediately gained his normal hearing back.

Shortly after, a patient with heart problems visited D. D. Palmer. He adjusted the patient's back, and the patient's heart problems disappeared. After these two events, D. D. Palmer began a systematic examination of the nervous system's role on human health. This was the beginning of chiropractic.[109]

For more than a hundred years, it was believed that vertebrae that were out of position mechanically pushed on nerves. Irritation in the nervous system was created, and it could influence the central nervous system, the peripheral nervous system, and the patient's ability to maintain homeostasis. Furthermore, it was believed that adjusting these vertebrae back to their normal position would recover nerve function and homeostasis. In the absence of better evidence, this explanation model was practiced both in clinics around the world and chiropractic educational institutions.

Over the past fifteen to twenty years, research has shown that the hypothesis of D. D. Palmer and his son B. J. Palmer was fundamentally correct. However, today we have a more accurate neurophysiological explanation model of what occurs in comparison to the previous mechanical explanation model.

Let me give you some updated scientific insight into the neurological mechanisms of chiropractic. We have previously stated that the brain and the central nervous system are essential when it comes to how we function and experience things. The brain is plastic and continuously changes depending on the kind of information it receives from our five classic senses (sight, smell, taste, hearing, and touch).[110]

This is thoroughly highlighted previously in this book. Based on scientific evidence, we see that specific chiropractic adjustments of the spine influence mechanoreceptors (pressure and touch) and nociceptors (pain) around the joints in the spine. This further results in the change of signals to the peripheral nervous system and the central nervous system, including a range of different areas of the brain. We will look closer at how an adverse function of the spinal column influences sensory receptors in and around the spinal column, which influences how the brain interprets our inner reality.

I will give you a small challenge. Place your hand somewhere behind your back without touching your back. Which of your five senses (sight, smell, taste, hearing, and touch) do you use to tell exactly where your hand is placed? You can't see it, you can't smell it, you can't taste it, you can't hear it, and you can't touch it.

To be able to answer the question we have to add a new sense called proprioception (joint sense). Proprioception is crucial in understanding how our body and mind cooperate. It is crucial in understanding chiropractic, and it is an important part of explaining the difference between chiropractic and conventional medicine (based on only five senses).

In addition to the central nervous system being located in the spinal column, sensory receptors are located in the passive structures around the joints and are also tightly packed in the small muscles around the spinal column (paraspinal musculature). These tiny little sensors react under strain (movement) in the musculature and send important information to the brain based on movement.

These small sensors act as the brain's eyes. They tell you exactly where in the room your arms, legs, and body are located at any point in time. These are the sensors that allow you to close your eyes and still be able to place your index finger on the tip of your nose without missing. This is called proprioception or joint sense. New research shows how the spinal column influences our senses and the way the brain perceives what is happening in the body.[111]

When the brain cannot interpret exactly what is happening in the body, it will send poor messages to the muscles and other structures.[112] It has been proven that some muscles have an extremely large amount of strain receptors. Due to this, many believe that these muscles' primary function is to send important sensory information to the brain, rather than providing movement.[113] [114] [115] [116]

When the spine does not move normally, the paraspinal muscles will move less and will provide you with a lack of information. I have previously highlighted how the brain guesses if it does not receive the normal amount of information. The brain will guess based on what you have previously experienced. Heidi Haavik uses a nice analogy in order to understand this in her book, *The Reality Check*. If you have lived in the same house for a long time, you know your way around the house. If there is a power outage during the night, you will probably be able to maneuver your way through the house to find the fuse box, even if you can't see.

Imagine that one of your children left a tricycle standing in the hallway that leads to the fuse box, which you did not notice before the power outage. What will happen? You will probably fall and hurt yourself. This is a likely explanation model of what happens when the brain does not receive accurate information from the rest of the body. When the brain does not receive information, it will guess based on previous knowledge and experiences.

In other words, sensory information from the spine is viewed as having an important function in how our inner reality is created, thus determining the type of response the body initiates. The greater the lack of "input" is, the greater the lack of "output" will be.

The body can be seen as a symphony orchestra, and the brain is the conductor that ensures that everyone is coordinated in order for everything to go smoothly.

These findings have led to a new chiropractic hypothesis. This hypothesis states that the brain's plastic ability to adjust itself detrimentally occurs when incoming signals from the spine are interrupted due to improper functioning in one or more joints in the spine.

The hypothesis states furthermore that a specific chiropractic adjustment can normalize the function of the dysfunctional joint, so the brain can adjust itself again in a fortunate way.

An improper function in the spine that leads to nerve irritation and changes in the associated soft tissue is called a subluxation.

"The vertebral subluxation's nerve interference causes an aberration in the flow of mental impulses from the brain cell to tissue cell, thus impairing normal function and altering the body's organic and physiological response to its environment".[117]

A subluxation will often include tenderness, poor mobility, and tight muscles around the joints.

The main goal for a chiropractor is to recover normal functioning in the musculoskeletal and nervous system when a subluxation arises. Adjustments (specific joint correction) are most often used. Research shows that there is a change in EMG activity in the paraspinal musculature due to an adjustment of the spinal column.[118] [119]

This is meaningful in relation to information that travels to the brain. Based on this, it is believed that a successful adjustment can lead to better communication between the brain, the body, and the body's outer environment.

In addition to subluxation's possible influence on sensory information from the spine to the brain, subluxation also influences how the brain responds to other sensory information.[120] For example, when you move your arm or leg, your brain must also take into consideration information coming from you spine in order to ensure stability and balance as you move. Studies show that chiropractic adjustments can influence joint senses. This refers to which position the joint is in at any point in time.[121]

I will give a clinical example. A soccer player at the highest level in Norway visited me because of acute low back pain. His team was supposed to play an important Europe League match a few days later. We worked intensively to get his back into proper shape. The player thought that his back felt okay while training the day before the match and decided to play the match. Not long after the match began, he completely missed a simple kick. Later on in the game, he sprained his ankle. Was it random? I think this happened because there was still a disruption of nerve signals from the spine. The brain was not 100 percent sure in which position the foot was, leading to a missed kick in the first half and the sprained ankle later in the game.

Research also shows that patients with lower back problems abnormally recruit posture-stabilizing muscles.[122]

The deep stomach muscles are an important part of the core musculature that stabilizes the back. It is important that stabilizing muscles take action before we, for example, lift our arms. This is to make sure that the body is stable. A study published in the *Journal of Manipulative and Physiological Therapeutics* in 2006 involving ninety young asymptomatic men showed that seventeen participants didn't activate stomach muscles before lifting up their arms.[123] They were retested six months later, and the results were the same. The examination findings showed that these participants had an impaired function of the joints between the sacrum and the ilium. After only one chiropractic treatment where the sacroiliac joint was adjusted, a 40 percent improvement in the activation of stomach muscles was observed before arms were raised.

An abnormal recruitment of posture-stabilizing muscles is not only found in patients with lower back pain. Studies show that this also applies to other conditions, such as knee pain.[124]

These findings are supported by other studies that show that improper functioning of the spine leads to a disturbance of the brain's interpretation of what is happening in the rest of the body.[125]

Until now, we have seen how a dysfunction of the spinal column changes information sent to the brain. The changing information to the brain can lead to unfavorable interpretations of the inner reality. This can lead to a changed response from the brain, such as poor control of the body in regards to pain and a reduced functioning ability.

It is universally accepted that pain in the left shoulder is a frequent indicator of a heart attack. This is a good example of how a heart attack is the cause of the brain's improper interpretation of incoming signals. There is nothing wrong with the shoulder.

This also shows that signals from an organ can influence the brain's interpretation of what is going on in the musculoskeletal system. This effect goes both ways and is called the somato-visceral reflex. "Somato" means body, whereas "viscera" means organ.

If we proceed with this explanation, which is widely accepted within conventional medicine, we should also believe that a dysfunction in the spinal column could lead to changing signals from the brain to other organs.

The study of pain mechanisms has led to a wider understanding of how chiropractic influences both the musculoskeletal system and the autonomous nervous system through the influence of the central nervous system.

In fact, the first fifty years of chiropractic existence was not about biomechanical neck and back pain at all. Chiropractic grew substantially after the flu epidemic in 1918. Chiropractors focused on the nervous system and innate intelligence to help people adapt to the environment.

In 2012, Coronado et al. could show that chiropractic adjustments of the spine influenced the dorsal root ganglia, which is a part of the central nervous system. The study also showed that a chiropractic adjustment of the neck led to decreased sensitivity both in the neck and in the lower back. This supports that an adjustment influences the central nervous system and that it does not just have a local effect on the peripheral nervous system.[126]

A study by Reed et al. in 2004 indicates that chiropractic adjustments of the spine reduce pain by influencing the thalamus (part of the brain), whereas mobilization does not seem to have the same effect.[127]

Mohammadian et al. conducted a study in 2004 that showed that adjustments of the spine influence nociceptors (pain) and mechanoreceptors (pressure and touch) at the level of a joint, leading to changes in the central nervous system on the brain stem level and/or cerebral level.[128]

In 2014, Gay et al. showed that adjustments of the thoracic spine led to direct and measurable effects of several areas of the central nervous system (limbic part of the cortex, insular cortex, motor cortex, amygdala, somatosensory cortex, and periaqueductal gray).[129]

Brain Region	Function
Cingulate Cortex	Emotions, learning, motivation, memory
Insular Cortex	Consciousness, homeostasis, perception, motor control, self-awareness, cognitive function
Motor Cortex	Voluntary movements

Amygdala Cortex	Memory, decision making, emotional reactions
Somatosensory Cortex	Proprio and mechanoreception, touch, temperature, pain of the skin, epithelium, skeletal muscle, bones, joints, internal organs, and cardiovascular systems
Periaqueductal Gray	Ascending and descending spinothalamic tracts carrying pain and temperature fibers

Table 3.1

In 2007, a study by Dickholtz et al. supported that chiropractic can influence different systems in the body.[130] This was an RCT, which looked at the effect a specific chiropractic adjustment of the upper neck (atlas) had on patients with high blood pressure. The study concluded that the normalization of the atlas's function is connected to a pronounced and lasting reduction in blood pressure. The result was the same as that with treatment combining two blood pressure-lowering medicines.

This study is a landmark for chiropractic, since the study received a bit of press coverage. At the same time, critics did not have anything to criticize within the study because the study was conducted on the evidence movement's own terms.

In the *Chiropractic Journal of Australia* in 2009, PL Rome PL analyzed nearly five hundred different studies that looked at the type of impact the spine can have on different organs.[131] The study has over 1,100 references. The study includes the visceral system, the immune system, the endocrine system, and different cognitive functions. In this study, Rome also pointed out that it is meaningless to attempt to classify different diseases since all conditions have a neurological component.

He writes, "There have been attempts to classify conditions under the manipulation of the spine in type M (muscle and skeletal diseases) and type O (organ diseases). If there would be any category at all, all conditions should come in under type N (neurological diseases) since all diseases have a neurological component."

The body or the heart's adaptability can be measured by looking at the way the heart works over time. This examination is called heart rate variability. Heart rate variability analyzes the balance between the peripheral nervous system (PNS) and the central nervous system (CNS) by looking at the heart's frequency behavior over time.

This type of analysis of the heart has been used as a measure of physical condition. New studies also indicate that this can be an important tool to reveal and follow disease processes or reduced functional ability. Reduced heart rate variability is seen in context with increased mortality, depression, diabetes, air pollution, disturbed cognitive function, and reduced memory. An increasing amount of evidence through studies conducted from different professions show that HRV can be used to evaluate the body's adaptability and autonomous nervous system.

A study from 2006 looked at the effect of chiropractic treatment on HRV and pain. The study collected data before and after the treatment of 625 patients divided among ninety-six chiropractic clinics. Of the total patients, 132 were followed up over a four-week period. The authors of the study write, "The group that received chiropractic treatment showed a significant improvement in HRV, both after a simple treatment and after treatment during a four-week period. The control group showed no significant improvement."[132]

The absence of pain is not necessarily equal to good health. Two studies show that improper functions persist even after a state of pain has improved.[133]

Instead of thinking that pain leads to dysfunction, this can be reversed where dysfunction causes pain.[134] This is of significance when it comes to how you perceive your own health, but it is also of significance for the therapist. Should a therapist only treat pain, or should the therapist also treat dysfunctions without pain? Most people are taught that the absence of pain equals good health, while pain equals problems. Unfortunately, many also "cheat" or fool themselves by resorting to painkillers as the only means of removing the pain. Painkillers will never do anything about the cause of pain! Research shows that you can walk around with dysfunctions without the presence of pain. An example from my clinical work is when I see considerable wear (degeneration) on an X-ray, and the patient only reports recent pain.

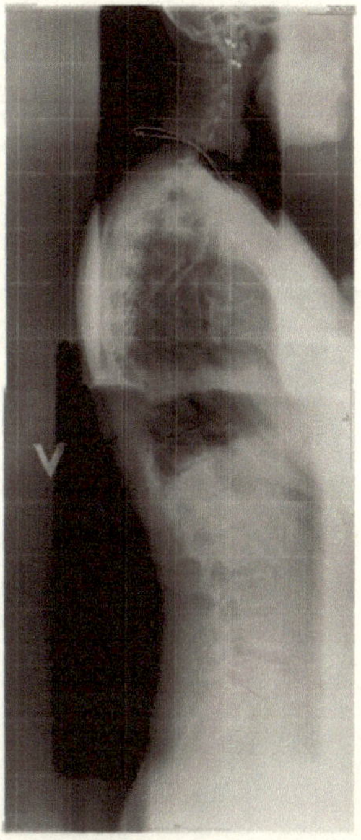

Figure 3.6. L5/S1 (lower disc in the Lumbar
spine) is significantly degenerated.

Degeneration is a result of dysfunction over time. Degeneration does not happen overnight or over a few weeks, but over years. A common scenario is when a patient comes to the clinic with acute lower back pain that arose acutely when the patient bent down to pick up a piece of paper from the floor. The X-ray reveals considerable degeneration of a specific segment (between two vertebrae). The back should of course handle picking up the piece of paper from the floor. We are talking about the last straw that broke the camel's back or the drop that caused the beaker to overflow.

In a treatment situation, it can be challenging to recommend further treatment based on dysfunction when the pain is gone. I do not want to be accused of recommending further treatment based on my income and not examination findings. The practitioner must show good ethical morality, while the patient must trust the practitioner.

A literature study by Hannon in 2004, where keywords such as "asymptomatic," "normal," "pain-free," "healthy" and "free from physical injury" were used, showed that chiropractic adjustments of subluxations led to measurable health benefits, regardless of the presence of pain.[135] The author concludes that there is a sufficient amount of evidence that supports that chiropractic can have a healthy effect on people without pain. Furthermore, the author concludes that there is plausible reason to claim that chiropractic can provide good health effects to all functions in the body and that chiropractic could potentially lead to good long-term health effects. Improvement in functioning among asymptomatic individuals, followed by chiropractic intervention, can be measured objectively without the use of invasive methods.

Posture

Proper posture and being aware of one's own body through a natural movement pattern was heavily emphasized during my education in Mensendieck physiotherapy in Oslo, Norway. The foundation of Mensendieck is good posture. A biomechanical model was used to argue why good body posture is important. The model also insinuated that this also could have positive effects beyond the purely biomechanical. Perhaps it is surprising that many chiropractors are equally concerned about good postures as physiotherapists. I believe that chiropractic has taken posture even a step further by looking at the neurological explanation model of the importance of having a good posture. Good posture is a key component for optimal health. How we adapt and behave to gravity is essential for our health and development.

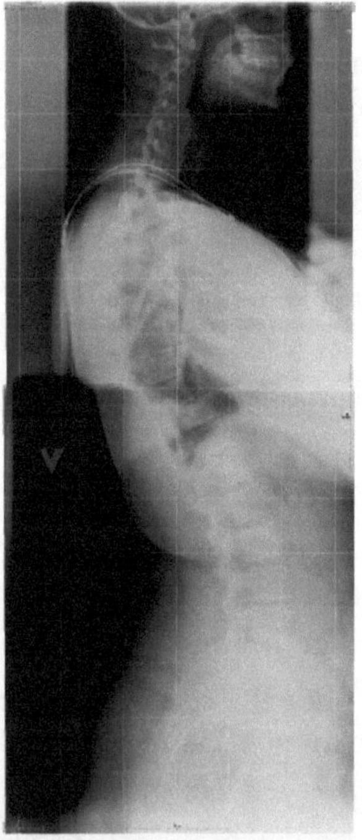

Figure 3.7. Slumped posture where the pelvis is pushed too far forward, the thoracic spine is rounded, and there is a forward head carriage, leading to a reversed neck curve. A typical EMG finding in such a patient will show lack of muscle tension in the lower back and buttocks and too much tension in the thoracic spine and neck.

Studies show that good posture can lead to different desired physiological changes:

- *Reduced fatigue and increased alertness* – Correction of forward head carriage may lead to reduced pain, tension, and stiffness in the neck, jaw, shoulders, and back, in addition to reduced fatigue and increased alertness.[136]
- *Increased confidence* – A good posture can cause hormonal changes that lead to improved self-confidence.[137] Arnette and fellow researchers indicate in their 2012 study that posture influences both our cognitive and emotional state.[138]
- *Improved self-evaluation* – Brinol and others showed in their 2009 study that good body posture could lead to a more positive self-image and positive thoughts, while poor body posture leads to more negative thoughts and a negative self-image.[139]

Studies also show that poor body posture can lead to various adverse physiological changes in the body:

- *Reduction of gray matter in the brain* – A study by Apkarian from 2004 showed that people with chronic low back pain experienced a ten to twenty times larger reduction of gray matter than those without low back pain.[140] Gray matter consists of nerve cell bodies and is partly involved in muscle control, seeing, hearing, speaking, memory, emotions, decision making, and so on. It was commonly found that individuals with poor posture have chronic low back pain.
- *Impaired heart and lung capacity* – A protruding head can lead to as much as a 30 percent reduction in lung capacity. A reduced lung capacity can be seen in relation to cardiovascular disease.[141]
- *Change in blood pressure and heart rate* – Increased tension in the neck musculature influences the solitary tract (part

of the brain), which plays an important role in regulating heart rate and blood pressure.[142]

- *Increased resistance in air passages* – Patients with asthma often have poor posture, which leads to the shortening of the musculature involved in breathing.[143]
- *An early death* – Increased thoracic kyphosis (slumped back) is connected to an earlier death among older men and women.[144] A more recent study published by Kado shows that an increased thoracic curve among older women gave a significantly greater chance of premature death, independent of parameters like osteoporosis.[145]
- *Increased risk of heart attack* – A study published in 2006 show that a 3-centimeter reduction in height among older men resulted in a 63 percent greater chance of heart attack. The same study concluded that men on average lose 1.67 centimeters in height during their lifetime.[146] This leads to a 42 percent increased risk of a heart attack.
- *Increased tendency of falling among the elderly* – There is a correlation between a slumped posture and an increased tendency to fall among the elderly. A slumped posture leads to decreased stability and balance among the elderly.[147]
- *Lower back pain* –Poor posture can lead to altered activation of the lumbar musculature and further to lumbar pain.[148] Another study supports this by showing patients with lumbar pain use other muscles to hold themselves upright.[149]

If you are skeptical of these studies, you can easily perform a few practical experiments that demonstrate the importance of a good body posture.

Sit down and slouch to make your back curved. Breathe in as deeply as you can. Notice how it feels to breathe. Straighten up your body and raise your chest upwards and forward. Now take a deep breath. Doesn't it feel much easier to breathe?

Push your head as far forward as you can. While your head is in this protruding position try to rotate or bend your head sideways as far as possible to each side. Balance your head over your shoulders. Now attempt the same movements. Was it easier this time?

Bend your head backwards or push your head as far forward as you can. Now try to swallow. Is it difficult? Elderly people with an extreme kyphotic posture often have their heads in this position. Do you think it might influence their appetite?

There is little doubt that a good posture is important for good health. But a good posture is still not enough. "A life in motion" is the slogan of the Norwegian Chiropractic Association. Having good posture does little good without being physically active. When a former colleague of mine was asked which position is the best way to sit, he always answered, "It is your next one." I can describe an ergonomically correct seated position for you, but I wouldn't want you to sit in this position for too long without moving. This applies to standing as well. Standing in the same position for an entire day is not better than sitting in the same position for an entire day. We need variety and movement. Movement gives the brain sensory motor information, which is essential for living. I have previously talked about the importance of being in homeostasis. The cerebellum is a center for homeostasis and has an important function in terms of movement.

Nothing on earth with intelligence remains motionless. When a child is born, it is born with primitive reflexes. These movements send sensory motor information to the brain. The brain can then process the information and send appropriate signals back to the body. The signals will develop the brain in terms of not only motor skills, but also cognitive skills. Without these innate primitive reflexes, infants would not be able to move, and the brain's development would be stunted. This applies throughout life. Health is perishable, and you must take care of it every single day of your life.

The art of practicing (chiropractic)

Treatment of human beings can never become more than an "educated guess." Experience plays an essential role in this process. As a practitioner, I believe that we should be rooted in philosophical and scientific principles, sprinkled with personal judgment and a good "gut feeling." I define gut feeling as a series of sensations too small to stand out on their own, but together strong enough to give an intuitive feeling of what to do. It gives an indication of whether something is right or wrong. A gut feeling is not something that randomly comes out of nowhere. As a practitioner, this can be called clinical intuition or the sixth sense (seventh sense if we include proprioception as the sixth sense). Snap judgments are accurate because intuition doesn't need processing by the conscious mind. This might possibly influence me to adjust a patient from the right side instead of the left side. I might adjust the joint from below instead of from above. Or I might adjust just one segment despite findings indications that four different segments are in trouble. My gut feeling might influence me to hold back an adjustment although there were examination results present, to further refer the patient to more examinations, or to advise the patient to come three times a week instead of one. No study will ever tell me exactly what to do every single time.

We have been taught that reason and the conscious mind is superior to intuition and the subconscious mind. Reason is much slower than intuition. Intuition doesn't judge; reason does. Still, reason is often used to justify intuition. Mrs. Petersen who is ninety years old and has pain in her thoracic spine can turn out completely different from twenty-four-year-old Mr. Olsen with the same type of pain. I might suspect a heart attack or a compression fracture in Mrs. Petersen, whereas I might suspect a subluxation or a stuck rib in Mr. Olsen. Both examinations and treatment will be very different. Even if my examination suggests the same findings in these two cases, treatment and treatment plan will be different.

The amount of force and adjustment techniques will be different. The frequency of treatment will be different. Both the short- and long-term prognosis will be different. The communication will be different. The ergonomic advice and guidance in regards to their treatment and exercises will most likely be different. All of these points are examples of the art of practicing, which is unfortunately drowning in the evidence-based practice of today.

We generally agree that the nervous system ultimately controls all bodily processes. It controls the gastrointestinal system, immune system, cardiovascular system, musculoskeletal system, the endocrine system, and so on.

I have argued thoroughly that our sensory experience or interpretation of incoming signals controls which physical measures the body initiates. I have also thoroughly highlighted that chiropractic influences both the incoming signals and outgoing signals through the stimulation of the nervous system. Chiropractic influences different parts of the brain and various parts of both the central and peripheral nervous systems. These areas control emotion, learning, motivation, memory, consciousness, homeostasis, perception, motor control, attention, cognitive functions, voluntary movements, decision making, touch, temperature, pain, muscle, bone, internal organs, the cardiovascular system, and more. Chiropractic should, therefore, be recognized for far more than treating back pain.

A chiropractor doesn't repair anything. A chiropractor does not treat diseases. Chiropractic is based on the concept that we are created to live a good and healthy life. A chiropractor emphasizes that nerve signals should travel without interference, so that the body can take care of itself and show its full potential. This is in line with my fundamental philosophy—we are created for health and wellness.

4

The Art of Living

Most people would say happiness is one of their main goals in life. When asked about what makes them happy, many will list marriage, children, and money.

Well, if you have children, especially for mothers, you will probably agree that this can be very challenging at times.

If you have married and still are married, you are soon to become a rarity.

Money can probably buy some kind of happiness to a certain degree of ensuring necessities, but when you get more of it, it often translates into a burden. Poverty can certainly lead to unhappiness, but more money does not necessary lead to happiness. People with lots of money are more often concerned about losing their fortune than they are about enjoying it. People who have won a huge amount of money on the lotto often say their life became troublesome after a while.

It seems when people achieve what they thought would make them happy, the dream was better than reality. A study done in Norway asked people about their favorite day of the week. Almost everyone put Friday on top of the list. The argument was that, on Friday, they had the entire weekend ahead. Interestingly, just a few put Saturday on top, and hardly anyone Sunday. It is not the actual weekend that makes us happy but the thought of it!

Measurements are reductions of experiences. Science rejects the subjective world because experiences are difficult to measure and are constantly changing.

If you love Mozart, and your spouse loves Justin Bieber, you will have different experiences when you listen to the two. Your ears will pick up the same wavelength, and the brain will receive the information in the same area, but you will have totally different experiences.

To experience happiness, your brain needs to send positive messages instead of negative ones.

What makes you happy? The ingredients are yours to create and maintain.

Take control of your own life and your future. Do not expect or wait for the government, health care system, or your health insurance to take care of your health and your future. You are solely responsible for your own life. Put yourself in the driver's seat and determine the way forward yourself. This requires active choices. Far too many are dissatisfied with their lives and future prospects but still choose to continue as before in the hope of something better. Einstein said, "Insanity is doing the same thing over and over again and expecting different results." I have explained earlier in this book how your future is already largely predetermined if you do the same things day after day. Failure and making mistakes is part of life. You can learn, grow, and develop when you correct flawed behavior.

Define your values and make a plan

You certainly have work instructions, tasks, and objectives if you have a job. The same certainly applies if you are an athlete. You do not become an elite athlete just because you want to.

If you want to go on a vacation, you probably have some ideas of where you want to go, how much it will cost, and how long you will stay. You collect information, book your trip, make sure that you and your family are free during this time, find someone to collect your mail and water your flowers while you are away, and so on and so forth.

What about your life in general? Have you thought about what it would take to fulfill your wishes and desires? Have you defined your values, goals, and the path toward your goals?

For example, consider these questions:

> What kind of family do you want to be a part of?
> What kind of social circle would you like?
> What type of employment do you want?
> How would you like your financial situation to be?
> How would you like to spend your spare time?
> What beliefs do you have?
> How often and how long would you like your vacation to be?
> Are weekends off important to you?

Dreams are important. Any goal you set begins with a dream. Visualize your dreams and act as if they have already happened. In order to achieve this, you need to accumulate a desire to achieve your dreams. It is your choice to choose your dreams. Do not let others do it for you.

If you don't know what you want, how will you succeed? Think about a chicken trying to poke a hole in its shell as it comes into the world. If someone helps it to pick open the hole, the hatchling will rarely survive. If you wait for someone to poke a hole in your shell, you will most likely not succeed. You are solely responsible for your own future.

I have been blessed to witness the hatching of baby turtles. The marine biologist who worked on the island said that, when turtles hatched, it was particularly important that they found their own way from the sandy beach where they hatched and down to the sea. Only in this way would they be able to come back to their place of origin to lay their eggs and contribute to the growth of the population.

I find that there are few people who have thought about their basic premises in order to be happy. Too many people walk around dissatisfied with life and complain about everything and everyone. I think many live a subconscious life. If you remember that most of our subconscious life is downloaded through observation of others, you will understand that you live your life dictated by those you have observed. I also think many have certainly not prioritized their values, and how can you really prioritize your values if you do not know what to prioritize?

I will give you a simple example.

John Doe is forty-five years old and lives with his wife, three children and two dogs. He is a CEO in a large company. He works twelve-hour shifts and often travels for business on the weekends. He has two directorships and is the leader in the local residents' association. His family is extremely well off financially. He is also physically active and exercises five times a week and is every now and then participating in triathlon competitions. In addition, he plays golf as often as he can.

When John Doe is asked to set up a priority list of what is important to him and what makes him happy in life, he emphasizes that time with his family is the most important. He explains how happy he is when he can spend time with his children as he watches them play, laugh, and grow. He ranks spending time with friends as number two. Further down the list, he mentions career and finances. Would this person be happy with his life?

John Doe's situation would have been quite different if his list was turned upside down. Remember previously that your own perception of your external reality determines your inner reality.

Remember the study from 2015 that showed that stress is not harmful as long as you are happy and thrive with stress.

My advice is to use time to go through the basic questions that will make you and your family happy. Back to where we started. If you have a solid philosophy, it is easier to choose an appropriate action in order to achieve well-being and reach your goals. Be honest with yourself. It is important that you do not answer these questions based on what you think is expected of you or what others want to hear. This is extremely difficult. Remember that 95 percent of who we are as human beings is determined by our unconscious mind and is downloaded through observing others. Your basic questions should be answered by your conscious mind. Ask open questions. I sometimes play around with the idea that it would be exciting to live with the motor skills and conscious mind of an adult and, at the same time, have the pure unconscious mind of a newborn child. How would I have sensed the world and what would have been important to me?

Also, remember that life is dynamic, and the goals that you set today are not necessarily applicable in ten years. Be tough and honest. Create new goals and new plans in order to achieve your new targets. Remember that your journey toward your goal is equally as important as the goal itself. Most of your time will be spent on your journey. Also remember that the dream often seems to be better than reality. If you have fulfilled your dream but have experienced that the dream was not what you expected, create new dreams.

The first time you did something perfectly is not because you did the exact same thing repeatedly. You have done something different, and that is why this particular time was different from the previous ones. You will not be able to repeat this perfect happening because every situation is different. You must constantly adapt to your environment.

Do not try to look for the ultimate answers. If they existed, life would be finite, meaning no further development. Think about your life as a river. There will be calm parts, and there will be wild parts.

Your ride in your river has infinite possibilities, but I can assure you that the exact same moment will never repeat itself.

I learned an important principle from a coach. The coach called this the "bouncer" principle. If you have taken the time to think through your values, it becomes much easier to exclude people and situations that are not consistent with your values. It is much harder to kick someone/something out of your life than to let that person or thing in. Many people who have a problem with saying no will recognize this. You do not have to deal with this if you have defined your values ahead of time. Just like the "bouncer," you can refuse entry to people or situations that are not consistent with your values.

If you don't want to be overweight, you probably recognize that it is much easier to avoid putting on weight in the first place than it is to lose it.

The same holds true for depression. It is easier to develop healthy thought processes than it is to work your way out of a depression.

You have probably noticed that you feel energetic around certain people, while it feels that energy is being drained when you hang around others. You may have noticed that someone in your social circle unconsciously is always complaining, criticizing. and speaking negatively. You may also have noticed how easy it is to be drawn into complaining and criticism. Hearing others complaining is almost as harmful as complaining yourself. Remember that your thoughts matter. Your thoughts decide your internal chemical state. Passive complaining is like passive smoking. By applying the "bouncer" principle, you can consciously spend more time with those who give you positive energy and less time with those who steal your energy.

Be – do – have

My nine-year-old daughter used to promise to behave *if* she got to have or do something that she wanted. I explained to her that it does not work that way. The "reward" will come afterward, not beforehand. If she is kind and does good things, good things will happen to her.

Most of us in the Western world today have more material possessions than previous generations ever had. Many of us have more time to do what we want, yet it seems that we are becoming more dissatisfied, stressed, and unhappy. We constantly hear about more people with psychological problems, such as stress, anxiety, fear, failure, depression, and the like. We use more and more medication to curb these problems. An increasing number of people are seeking escapism.

If external circumstances determine whether or not you are happy, then external circumstances control how you feel.

Far too many in today's society begin at the wrong end. We require higher wages first. Then we will consider making more of an effort. We will behave appropriately *if* this or that happens. We will be happy *if* we have just the things we want.

Being happy must come from within. If you are happy and satisfied, you will automatically do positive things that happy and satisfied people do, and you are likely to have the things you want in life. You determine how you want your life to be and the way you feel. "Cause and effect" is a known scientific term. However, imagine if you could replace the word "cause" with "causing." "Causing an effect"—wouldn't that be much better? Again remember how your mind controls your inner reality. The thoughts that you allow your mind to have are a reflection of your life. We are generally always correct when we believe that we can or cannot do something. You will almost certainly fail if you expect to do so. By changing your expectations, you are simultaneously changing your behavior.

Next time you are dreading something, consider this; you probably do not fear the situation itself but, rather, your own feelings in that particular situation. As I have pointed out, you can change your thoughts, which in turn influences your emotions.

Doesn't it sound wonderful to be able to control your thoughts and, by doing so, decide the kind of life you lead?

You can achieve what you focus on.
You can choose how you behave.
You can choose how you will feel.
You can choose whom you attract.
You can choose how you will react to what you are experiencing.
You are the driver of your car, and you decide where to drive.

People and their thoughts consist of energies, and similar energies attract each other. This is about "The law of attraction." For example, good thoughts, love, and joy lead to good health, while anger, grief, depression, and jealousy lead to disease. Most people are not aware that thoughts have a frequency and can be measured. Thoughts are energies.

In the chapter on quantum physics, I explained how the smallest particles that exist are energy. I also explained how this energy collapses and becomes visible or material by observation. It follows that thoughts become things.

As previously mentioned, you can choose what you want to observe and, thus, have an impact in influencing your future. Look at yourself as a magnet with opportunities to attract desirable future events. If you live as if what you want already happened, then your body will emit energies accordingly. Further, this follows the principle "like attracts like."

I find that this law is often misinterpreted. You can not be passive and think that good thoughts, God, Allah, or other external forces alone will lead you to what you want.

Look at your life like a GPS. If you visit a friend who has just moved to a new address, it is not enough to just plot the new address into your GPS and wait to arrive. If the vehicle is in park, you will remain in the same place. Put the car into gear and start driving. If you are driving in the wrong direction, your GPS tells you that you are driving in the wrong direction. The same applies if you have your basic philosophy, values, and goals set in place. You still need to start your journey. Unfavorable choices will appear during the journey. Your basic philosophy will guide you to the right choices.

If you stray from these values, your built-in GPS will tell you that you are on the wrong course. Then you will be able to turn around. The path will appear as you travel along. Many expect to see their goal clearly throughout the entire journey and receive constant clear confirmation that they are on the right path. Your final destination, your friend's new house, will appear equally unclear when you are a thousand meters away as when you started your journey. This is the same with your goals in life as well. If your journey had been clear the entire way, your fate would have been predetermined. You would have acted based on Newton's principles, where A leads to B, and B leads to C, and so on.

You will only notice that you have reached your destination when you have reached it.

We have seen that you can consciously make efforts to influence your blood pressure. Do you think the same could be possible to achieve with chronic diseases, cancer, and similar health-related problems?

William James said, "Human beings can alter their lives by altering their attitudes of mind."

It sounds almost too good to be true that you can determine how your own life will be, but why do so many people fail?

According to research, we complain on average once a minute during a conversation. Trevor Blake, author of *Three Simple Steps*, says there is a reason for the complaining. "Nothing unites people more strongly than a common dislike. The easiest way to build friendships and communicate is through something negative." Some point out that the negative is a part of evolution as being a self-defense or a survival instinct. Remember how I previously explained the adverse consequences Darwin's "survival of the fittest" has on us as human beings. If you don't master your enemy, your enemy will master you.

Many people are taught to focus on problems, mistakes, what is not there, what should have been, or what one should have done. We have lost sight of all the good and wonderful qualities in ourselves.

Nursing a negative emotion is effective on blocking positive emotions. If you say to yourself that you are not as fit anymore or your brain is not as sharp as it was, you are training your brain to live up to your diminished expectations. Low expectations will lead to low achievements.

Be honest with yourself. How do you feel about yourself? Do you like who you are? Are you a good version of yourself? Do you think of yourself as a good, happy, and successful person who contributes positively to the society we live in? How do you talk to yourself? If you talked to your best friend the same way you talk to yourself, would you still be friends?

In a society where access to information has become extremely extensive, we are constantly bombarded with problems and sad news. Next time you watch the news, count how many sad and terrible stories are presented in comparison to the amount of positive news. No wonder many struggle to think positively. We worry ourselves too much. Most of what we worry about will never happen or relates to things we can't influence.

"The reason why worry kills more people than work, is that more people worry than do work" (Robert Frost).

There are things you can do something about and things you can't do anything about. Use your energy on the first.

A good example is the weather. If you choose to live in Norway, you have to take into consideration our four seasons. Try to adjust instead of complaining. Find different things to enjoy about the different seasons. If you do not like winter, make it easier by buying a snowblower and warm clothes. Make the winter cozier by lighting candles or starting a fire in the fireplace. You can't do anything about the weather. You are only compromising yourself if you go around grumpy and complaining.

Do not let outside circumstances control you. Define your values and find a "bouncer" so that you do not run into someone/ something that degrades your quality of life. Being happy and joyful comes from within. It must come from who you are and what you feel about yourself. It has to do with your identity.

It strikes me that many people are satisfied with being mediocre. Here is a saying about it: "I have good news and bad news for you. The bad news is that you are going to struggle with this for the rest of your life. The good news is that you're going to get used to it!"

I hear almost weekly examples of this in my everyday practice. Typically, a patient enters with some type of acute pain. When I ask the patient how he or she is doing after a few consultations, I commonly hear, "Everything is going great. The acute pain is completely gone. Now I just have my usual pain." The patient is satisfied with mediocrity and accepts a pain that probably does not need to be there. Life should be about more than just survival.

The first step to being happy is to expect that change will happen.

We often find excuses and look to others who struggle, others who don't manage, a downturn in the market, and so on. Ask yourself then, Does anyone at all get it? Why can't this be me?

A person who finds excuses for everything will never succeed. You will fail if you excuse what you do and who you are. Turn excuses into opportunities. In order to change something, you have to have hope. Without hope and expectation, no change will occur. The moment you have a clear intention of a new future, this links to a positive feeling and causes the body to change. You are now no longer living in the past.

The aim of this book is for you as a reader to be able to make changes that lead to an improved quality in your life. I also know that probably only 5 to 10 percent will make a change due to receiving new information. In order to increase this percentage, you have to be motivated. The chance of change will then be greater. It turns out that of the greatest importance for achieving change is a direct experience. For those who are passionate about something, the passion is usually comes from having had an experience that they felt connected to. Remember the married couple having the conversation about a low-carb diet and health. The man had first read that this could be good for him, but he had also made the crucial next step of putting this into practice. When he experienced its effect on his health, he enthusiastically spread this information to others. As a reader of this book, you should create some concrete tasks based on what you wish to change so you can create an experience. For example, you can create something similar to the example below.

In February 2015, more than a thousand people attended a project, the Complaint Restraint Project run by Thierry Blancpain and Pieter Pelgrims, where participants were not allowed to complain for an entire month. Try it yourself and see how it affects your life. This is an experiment where you can prove to yourself how positive thoughts have a positive impact on your life. When life doesn't develop the way we want in my family, we use this practice. We call it happy month. In the complaint-free month we also have a jar to put money in, if some of us fail with a complaint or being negative. At the end, we do something nice with the money we put in the jar. Most often there is almost no money in the jar, and we have been rewarded with a happier month.

We think in pictures, not words

Negative thoughts often involve the word *not*. The brain can't interpret this word. Rather, it reinforces the following words, phrases, and ideas. Let's do a little experiment. *Do not* think of the number 4. Absolutely, do *not* think of a blue number 4. This blue number 4 is *not* flashing. It is difficult to envision anything else than a blue flashing number 4, isn't it?

Here is another simple experiment. Imagine that you are **not** allowed to scratch your head. If you manage to remain aware of **not** scratching your head, how long does it take before you begin to feel the need to scratch your head?

I have thus explained that your thoughts control your inner reality. I have further demonstrated through two simple experiments how this works in practice. The body perceives what *follows* the word *not*.

Think about the kind of impact this has on health or life in general. Joe Dispenza, DC, has traveled around the world interviewing a bunch of people who have experienced so-called medical miracles. This includes people who received a deadly diagnosis and were told that they only had a short period left to live. They somehow experienced a spontaneous inclination; all examinations checked out fine, and all trace of disease disappeared. Dispenza wanted to know more about the cause of these miracles. He says that the reason lies neither in belief nor in gender, ethnicity, skin color, or similar factors. He said that those who experienced medical miracles are often people who decided to continue living. This sounds self-explanatory, but most people with a fatal diagnosis will think differently. They think that they must *not* die. Remember what happens after the word "not"? The desire to live must be greater than the fear of dying.

Perhaps you have noticed that you become sick more easily if you think that you can't be sick at that particular moment?

We all have a wonderful opportunity to choose. Winners make good choices. Winners choose differently than do losers.

In a sports context, this should be a familiar phenomenon. The desire to win must be greater than the fear of losing. What do you think happens to an athlete who thinks, *I must not fall; I can't be nervous; we must not lose*?

Since the brain is unable to interpret the word "not," it is extremely important that we choose to focus on what we want to happen, not what we do not want to happen. Choosing is your choice.

If you find it difficult to think of what should *not* happen or maybe you are on the brink of getting a panic attack, then it might be a good exercise to think about something specific that can occupy your thoughts instead of thinking of what you do not want to happen. For example, begin by describing the objects around you and continue by counting these items. Sometimes this can effectively break the pattern of thinking about what you do not want to happen.

You could also put yourself on the outside as an observer. You will often get a different perspective. Try this: Look at a dog. Observe the dog and notice what you are thinking about. Now try to imagine you are the dog. What do you feel or think about now? Do you notice any difference?

Along with my advice of attempting a complaint-free month, how about going a month where you do not think about what you do not want to happen? You are only allowed to think about what you want to happen and, preferably, behave as if it has already happened. As a seed grows into a plant, your thoughts grow to become your reality.

"I will try" is a well- known phrase. By saying that you will try, you have already opened yourself up to fail. You say you will try because you do not believe. If you believe in what you say, you would say that you will, not that you will try. By trying, you attempt to force a result without believing in your ability to actually do it. Do not try! Either you do it or you do not. Chances for success will be much greater.

Live in the future, not in the past

It is more powerful to live in the future and not in the past if you want to create your own reality. This means that, if you behave as if something has happened, your body will produce an internal chemical composition as if it actually already happened. Think back to quantum physics, where you release yourself from time, place, and space. You should be grateful for whatever comes, not just for what has occurred. Most of us are grateful only after we have experienced something we appreciate. This also corresponds with the reverse order of be-do-have. If you follow this road, you will most likely not progress to the next step. You are, once again, back to the external environment, which you do not control, determining your fate and future.

It is also important to point out that you must believe in your dreams and desires. The subconscious part of your mind must believe in the conscious part because when you live in the present the unconscious part of the mind is your default program and essentially controls your actions.

You can change your unconscious mind

There are four ways to change your unconscious mind.

You can change it through hypnosis. Remember that this is a condition in which the brain operates in theta mode and can be changed.

Theta mode is the brain's work frequency right before you fall asleep. One suggestion is that every night before you are going to sleep, think about the positive experiences you had that day and what you were satisfied with. Many people do exactly the opposite. They think about what they should have done differently, what went wrong, what irritated them, or the stresses that they will face the next day.

If you have children, the last thing you can do before bedtime is to ask your child, what was the best part of his or her day? This will be a good habit for the rest of your child's life.

Repetition is another way to influence your subconscious mind. I wrote earlier about how driving a car transitioned from being a conscious act of learning to largely an unconscious act through repetition. For example, if you decide to have a complaint-free month, it could lead to good experiences, and you might want to try it for another month. Eventually, a complaint-free everyday becomes a part of your unconscious mind, where you focus on the good things rather than the bad.

A third way to change the unconscious mind is through special programs. These methods can be effective to change your downloaded programs in a short period of time.

This book will not deal with such programs.

The last way to change the unconscious mind unfortunately happens sometimes. Reprogramming can also happen through a severe trauma.

Without knowing for certain, I assume that many who were on Utøya, Norway, on July 22, 2011, where sixty-nine youngsters were massacred, experienced severe trauma that changed them. After this terrible incident, their subconscious mind has probably changed. What happened on 9/11 in New York is another example.

Start with yourself

For many people, it is easier to criticize and find faults in others than it is to look at themselves.

We must all begin with ourselves.

This becomes especially important when we know that 95 percent of our operative programs are downloaded through observations, primarily from the first six to seven years of life.

If you say one thing to a child but act differently, the child always notice what you do, not what you say. For example, there will be little effect on your child if you verbally tell your child he or she may not eat sweets while he or she sees you eating sweets. There is little effect on your children if you tell them that they use the iPad or watch TV too much, if you are doing the same. There is little effect on your children if you tell them not to be grumpy if you are grumpy. If you complain and focus on negative things, your child will probably adapt a similar behavior. Although you may not like it, you may have heard from others that you behave just like your mom or dad in certain situations. Statements such as "you are just like your father" or "that is just like something your mother would have done" are familiar statements to many.

Before you criticize others, always begin with yourself. If you walk around as a good example, you will probably affect others around you in a positive way.

You will never be as young as you are today. What are you waiting for?

"A new philosophy, a new way of life, is not given for nothing. It has to be paid dearly for and only acquired with much patience and great effort" (Fyodor Dostoyevsky).

It is easy to blame the media for our constant exposure to scandals and terrible news. I am not sure which came first, the chicken or the egg. Perhaps it lies in human nature that we want to hear about others who are worse off than we are. Maybe that is the reason media presents this type of news. If nobody were interested in this type of news, the media would probably not present it. In order to create a change, consumers must change their views. In the "old days," a farrier was on every street corner. Today, we find a pharmacy on every street corner. What is next? I hope it is something health related and not illness related. We have to begin with ourselves in order for this to happen.

On his deathbed, Albert Einstein said, "In the final analysis, it all comes down to one question—is the universe a friendly place? Your answer will determine the kind of life you lead."

References

1 MetLife Foundation, "What America Thinks: MetLife Foundation Alzheimer's Survey," study conducted by Harris Interactive, February 2011.

2 Fritjof Capra, *The Turning Point: Science, Society, and the Rising Culture* (New York: Bantam Books, 1983), 146.

3 http://www.reseptregisteret.no.

4 E. Calle, C. Rodriguez, et al., "Overweight, Obesity, and Mortality from Cancer in a Prospectively Studied Cohort of US Adults," *The New England Journal of Medicine* 348 (2003): 1625–38.

5 American Cancer Society, *Cancer Facts & Figures 2006*, Atlanta, GA: American Cancer Society, 2006; JM McGinnis and WH Foege. "Actual Causes of Death in the United States," *JAMA* 270 (1993): 2207–2212.

6 Dennis T. Jaffe, PhD, *Healing from Within* (New York: Simon & Schuster, Inc.), 15–17, 21, 28, XVII, 63, 25, XVI, 27, 56.

7 Centers for Disease Control and Prevention, *National Diabetes Fact Sheet: General Information and National Estimates on Diabetes in the United States*, 2005.

8 Centers for Disease Control and Prevention.

9 Gary Null et al., "Death by Medicine," *Life Extension Magazine*, August 1, 2006. http://www.webdc.com/pdfs/deathbymedicine.pdf.

10 B. Starfield, "Is US Health Really the Best in the World?" *JAMA* 284, no. 4 (July 26, 2000): 483–85.

11 B. Starfield, "Deficiencies in US Medical Care. *JAMA* 284, no. 17 (November 1 2000): 2184–85.

12 J1 Lazarou, BH Pomeranz, and PN Corey, "Incidence of Adverse Drug Reactions in Hospitalized Patients: A Meta-Analysis of Prospective Studies," *JAMA* 279, no. 15 (April 15, 1998): 1200–1205.

13 MA Ismail, "Drug Lobby Second to None: How the Pharmaceutical Industry Gets Its Way in Washington," *The Center for Public Integrity*, July 7, 2005.

14 Law, *Big Pharma: Exposing the Global Healthcare Agenda*, 2006.

15 R. A. Hayward et al., "Narrative Review: Lack of Evidence for Recommended Low-Density Lipoprotein Treatment Targets: A Solvable Problem," *Annals of Internal Medicine* 145 (2006): 520–530.

16 J Abramson and JM Wright, "Are Lipid-Lowering Guidelines Evidence-Based?" *The Lancet* 369 (2007): 168–169.

17 Capra, *The Turning Point*, 137–38.

18 O.T. Avery, C.M. MacLeod, M McCarty. "Studies on the chemical nature of the substance inducing transformation of pneumococcal types. Induction of transformation by a desoxyribosenucleic acid fraction isolated from pneumococcus type III", J Exp. Med., 79(1944), pp. 137-158.

19 D. Schmucker and J. C. Clemens, el al., "Drosophila DSCAM Is an Axon Guidance Receptor Exhibiting Extraordinary Molecular Diversity," *Cell* 101 (2000): 671–84.

20 Pray 2004; Silverman 2004.

21 Dawson Church, PhD, *Genie in Your Genes*.

22 Tina Rönn, Petr Volkov, C Davegårdh, T Dayeh, E Hall, AH Olsson, E Nilsson, A Tornberg, M Dekker Nitert, KF Eriksson, HA Jones, L Groop, and C Ling, "A Six Months Exercise Intervention Influences the Genome-Wide DNA Methylation Pattern in Human Adipose Tissue," *PLOS Genetics* 9 no. 6 (June 2013): e1003572, doi: 10.1371/journal.pgen.1003572. Epub June 27, 2013.

23 Pennisi, 2003; Pearson, 2003; Goodman, 2003.

24 Blaxter, 2003.

25 Blaxter, 2003; Celniker et al., 2002.

26 http://www.fhi.no/artikler/?id=101058, korrigert i 2014; HS Blix, K Landmark, R Selmer, and A Reikvam, Forskrivning av antihypertensive legemidler, 1975–2010; R. Selmer, HS Blix, K Landmark, and A Reikvam, "Choice of Initial Antihypertensive Drugs and Persistence Of Drug Use—A Four-Year Follow-Up of 78453 Incident Users," *Tidsskr Nor Laegeforen* 132, no. 10 (May 29, 2012): 1224–28; *European Journal of Clinical Pharmacology* 68, no 10. (October 2012): 1435–42.

27 Appenzeller, "Evolution: Test Tube Evolution Catches Time in a Bottle," *Science* 284, no. 5423 (June 25 1999): 2108.

28 John Snow, *On the Mode of Communication of Cholera* (London: J. Churchill, 1849).

29 Pasteur, Louis, *Comptes rendus, de l'Academie des Sciences* XC [On the Extension of the Germ Theory to the Etiology of Certain Common Diseases], trans. H. C. Ernst, (May 1880), 1033–44.

30 Robert Koch, "2 Die Aetiologie der Tuberkulose," *Mittheilungen aus dem Kaiserlichen Gesundheitsamt* (1884): 1–88; R Koch, "Ueber den augenblicklichen Stand der bakteriologischen Choleradiagnose," *J. Hyg. Inf.* 14 (1893): 319–33.

31 Virgil V. Strang, DC, PhC, *Essential Principles of Chiropractic* (Davenport, IA: Palmer College of Chiropractic, 1984), 11, 30.

32 B. J. Palmer, *As a Man Thinketh*, reproduced by Delta Sigma Chi Fraternity, 1988.

33 Liboff, 2004; Goodman and Blank, 2002; Sivitz, 2000; Jin et al., 2000; Blackman et al., 1993; Rosen, 1992; Blank, 1992; Tsong, 1989; and Yen-Patton et al., 1988.

34 McClare, 1974.

35 Larry Dossey, MD, *Prayer is Good Medicine* (New York: Harper-Collins, 1996), 55.

36 E. B. Harvey, "A Comparison of the Development of Nucleate and Non-Nucleate Eggs of *Arbacia punctulata*," *Biology Bullitin* 79 (1940): 166–87; M. K. Kojima; "Effects of D2O on Parthenogenetic Activation and Cleavage in the Sea Urchin Egg," *Development, Growth, and Differentiation* 1, no. 26 (1984): 61–71; B. H. Lipton, K. G. Bensch, and M. A. Karasek, "Microvessel Endothelial Cell Transdifferentiation: Phenotypic Characterization," *Differentiation* 46 (1991): 117–133.

37 Tsong, 1989.

38 MF Fraga, E Ballestar, MF Paz, S Ropero, F Setien, ML Ballestar, D Heine-Suñer, JC Cigudosa, M Urioste, J Benitez, M Boix-Chornet, A Sanchez Aguilera, C Ling, E Carlsson, P Poulsen, A Vaag, Z Stephan, TD Spector, YZ Wu, C Plass, And M Esteller, "Epigenetic Differences Arise during the Lifetime of Monozygotic Twins," *Proceeding of the National Academy of the Sciences of the United States of America* 102, no. 30 (July 26, 2005): 10604–10609, Epub July 11 2005.

39 Lipton et al., 1991.

40 Segerstrøm and Miller, 2004; Kopp and Rethelyi, 2004; McEwen and Lasky, 2002, McEwen and Seeman, 1999.

41 Dispenza, "You are the Placebo."

42 Takamatsu et al., 2003; Arnsten and Goldman-Rakic, 1998; Goldstein et al., 1996.

43 Keller, Litzelman, Wisk, et al., "Does the Perception that Stress Affects Health Matter? The Association with Health and Mortality," *Health Psychology* 31, no. 5 (September 2012): 677–84.

44 JP Jamieson, MK Nock, and WB Mendes, "Mind over Matter: Reappraising Arousal Improves Cardiovascular and Cognitive Responses to Stress," *Journal of Experimental Psychology: General* 141, no. 3 (August 2012): 417–22, doi: 10.1037/a0025719, Epub September 26, 2011.

45 Rhoshel K. Lenroot, Nitin Gogtay, Deanna K. Greenstein, Elizabeth Molloy Wells, Gregory L. Wallace, Liv S. Clasen, Jonathan D. Blumenthal, Jason Lerch, Alex P. Zijdenbos, Alan C. Evans, Paul M. Thompson, and Jay N. Giedd, "Sexual Dimorphism of Brain Developmental Trajectories during Childhood and Adolescence."

46 V. J. DiRita, "Genomics Happen," *Science* 289 (2000): 1488–89.

47 B. E. Schwarz, "Ordeal by Serpents, Fire and Strychnine," *Psychiatric Quarterly* 34 (1960): 405–429.

48 Kevin Crush, "Hotfoot It: Walking on Red-Hot Coals Is All about the Energy," *Grande Prairie Daily Herald Tribune*, June 17, 2005.

49 Lewis Mehl-Madrona, *Coyote Wisdom: The Power of Story in Healing* (Rochester, VT: Inner Traditions/Bear & Company, 2005), 37.

50 Cecil Adams, "Supermom: Could a mother actually lift a car to save her child?" *The Straight Dope*, January 20, 2006.

51 Angela Cavallo, 2006 (ref 5 kap 1).

52 Fratello F, Veniero D, Curcio G, et al., "Modulation of Corticospinal Excitability by Paired Associative Stimulation: Reproducebility of Effects and Intraindividual Reliability," *Clinical Neurophysiology* 117, no. 12 (2006): 2667–74; J Liepert, H Bauder, HR Wolfgang, WH Miltner, E Taub, and C Weiller, "Treatment- Induced Cortical Reorganization after Stroke in Humans," *Stroke* 31, no. 6 (June 2000): 1210–16; BJ Sessle, D Yao, H Nishiura, et al., "Properties and Plasticity Induced by Extensive Training Revealed by Transcranial Magnetic Stimulation in Human," *European Journal of Neuroscience* 21, no. 1 (2005): 259–66; M Tinazzi, M Valeriani, G Moretto, et al., "Plastic Interactions between Hand and Face Cortical Representation in Patients with Trigeminal Neuralgia: A Somatosensory-Evoked Potentials Study," *Neuroscience* 127, no. 3(2004): 769–76; T Weiss et al., "Rapid Functional Plasticity" in the Primary Somatomotor Cortex and Perceptual Changes after Nerve Block," *European Journal of Neuroscience* 20, no. 12 (December

2004): 3413–23; JN Sanes and JP Donoghue, "Plasticity and Primary Motor Cortex," *Annual Reviews Neuroscience* 23 (2000): 393–415; F Tye, A Boyadjian, and H Devanne, "Motor Cortex Plasticity Induced by Extensive Training Revealed by Transcranial Magnetic Stimulation in Human," *European Journal of Neuroscience* 21, no. 1 (2005): 259–66; A Kalin-Lang, L Sawaki, and LG Cohen. "Role of Voluntary Drive in Encoding an Elementary Motor Memory," *Journal of Neurophysiology* 93, no.2 (February 1, 2005): 1099–1103).

53   Tye et al. "Motor Cortex Plasticity Induced," 259–66; R. Nudo R, G. Miliken, W Jenkins, and M Merzenich. "Use-Dependent Alterations of Movement Representations in Primary Motor Cortex of Adult Squirrel Monkeys," *Journal of Neuroscience*16, no. 2 (January 15, 1996): 785–807; S Yahagi, Y Takeda, Z Ni, et al., "Modulation of Input-Output Properties of Corticospinal Tract Neurons By Repetitive Dynamic Index Finger Abductions," *Experimental Brain Research* 161, no. 2 (2005): 255–64; NN Byl, MM Merzenich, S Cheung, P Badenbaugh, SS Nagarajan, and WM Jenkins, "A Primate Model for Studying Focal Dystonia and Repetitive Strain Injury: Effects on the Primary Somatosensory Cortex," *Physical Therapy* 77, no. 3 (1997): 269–84; CI Renner, M Schubert, and H Hummelsheim, "Selective Effects of Repetitive Hand Movements on Intracortical Inhibition," *Muscle & Nerve* 31, no. 3 (March 2005): 314–320; M Schubert, E Kretzschmar, G Waldmann, and H Hummelsheim, "Influence Of Repetitive Hand Movements on Intracortical Inhibition," *Muscle & Nerve* 29, no. 6 (June 2004): 804–811; NN Byl and M Melnick, "The Neural Consequences of Repetition: Clinical Implications of a Learning Hypothesis," *Journal of Hand Therapy* 10, no. 2 (April–June 1997): 160–74; Weiss et al., "Rapid Functional Plasticity," 3413–23; JP Brasil-Neto, LG Cohen, A Pascual-Leone, FK Jabir, RT Wall, and M Hallett, "Rapid Reversible Modulation of Human Motor Outputs after Transient Deafferentation of the Forearm: A Study with Transcranial Magnetic Stimulation," *Neurology* 42, no. 7 (1992): 1302–1306; M Tinazzi, T Rosso, G Zanette, A Fiaschi, and SM Aglioti, "Rapid Modulation of Cortical Proprioceptive Activity Induced by Transient Cutaneous Deafferentation: Neurophysiological Evidence of Short- Term Plasticity across Different Somatosensory Modalities in Humans," *European Journal of Neuroscience* 18, no. 11 (2003): 3053–60; BA Murphy, H Haavik Taylor, SA Wilson, JA Knight, KM Mathers, and S Sshug, "Changes in Median Nerve Somatosensory Transmission and Motor Output Following Transient Deafferentation of the Radial

Nerve In Humans," *Clinical Neurophysiology* 114, no. 8 (2003): 1477–88; BA Murphy and N Dawson, "The Effects Of Repetitive Contractions and Ischemia on the Ability to Discriminate Intramuscular Sensation," *Somatosensory & Motor Research* 19, no. 3 (2002): 191–97; M Hallett, R Chen, U Ziemann, and LG Cohen, "Reorganization in motor cortex in Amputees and in Normal Volunteers after Ischemic Limb Deafferentation," *Electroencephalography & Clinical Neurophysiology – Supplement* 51 (1999), 183–87; Tinazzi M, Zanette G, Polo A, et al. "Transient Deafferentation in Humans Induces Rapid Modulation of Primary Sensory Cortex Not Associated with Subcortical Changes: A Somatosensory Evoked Potential Study. *Neuroscience Letters* 223, no. 1 (1997): 21–24; JP Brasil-Neto, J Valls-Sole, A Pascual-Leone, et al., "Rapid Modulation of Human Cortical Motor Outputs Following Ischaemic Nerve Block," *Brain* 116, pt. 3 (1993): 511–25; SF Cooke and TV Bliss, "Plasticity in the Human Central Nervous System," *Brain* 129, pt. 7 (2006): 1659–73; LG Cohen, U Ziemann, and R Chen, "Mechanisms, Functional Relevance and Modulation of Plasticity in the Human Central Nervous System," in W Paulus, M Hallett, PM Rossini, and JC Rothwell, eds., *Transcranial Magnetic Stimulation* (USA: Elsevier Science BV, 1999), 174–82.

54 Fabrizio Benedetti, Helen S. Mayberg, Tor D. Wager, Christian S. Stohler, and Jon-Kar Zubieta, "Neurobiological Mechanisms of the Placebo Effect," *The Journal of Neuroscience* 25, no. 45 (November 9, 2005): 10390–402, doi: 10.1523/JNEUROSCI.3458-05.2005.

55 Colloca and Benedetti, 2005; DG Finniss and F Benedetti "Mechanisms of the Placebo Response and Their Impact on Clinical Trails and Clinical Practice," *Pain* 114: 3–6.

56 A Hróbjartsson and PC Gøtzsche, "An Analysis of Clinical Trials Comparing Placebo with No Treatment," *New England Journal of Medicine* 344 (2001): 1594–602.

57 BE Wampold, ZE Imel, and T Minami. "The Placebo Effect: 'Relatively Large' and 'Robust' Enough to Survive Another Assault," *Journal of Clinical Psychology* 63, no. 4 (2007): 401–403.

58 JB Moseley Jr., NP Wray, D Kuykendall, K Willis, and G Landon, "Arthroscopic Treatment of Osteoarthritis of the Knee: A Prospective, Randomized, Placebo-Controlled Trial: Results of a Pilot Study," American Journal of Sports Medicine 24, no. 1 (January–February 1996): 28–34.

59 JB Moseley, K O'Malley, NJ Petersen, TJ Menke, BA Brody, DH Kuykendall, JC Hollingsworth, CM Ashton, and NP Wray, "A Controlled Trial of Arthroscopic Surgery for Osteoarthritis Of The Knee," *New England Journal of Medicine* 347, no. 2 (July 11 2002): 81 –88.

60 Raine Sihvonen, MD, Mika Paavola, MD, PhD, Antti Malmivaara, MD, PhD, Ari Itälä, MD, PhD, Antti Joukainen, MD, PhD, Heikki Nurmi, MD, Juha Kalske, MD, and Teppo LN Järvinen, MD, PhD, for the Finnish Degenerative Meniscal Lesion Study (FIDELITY) "Group Arthroscopic Partial Meniscectomy versus Sham Surgery for a Degenerative Meniscal Tear," *North England Journal of Medicine* 369 (December 26, 2013): 2515–24, doi: 10.1056/NEJMoa1305189.

61 S Vits, E Cesko, P Enck, U Hillen, D Schadendorf, and M Schedlowski, "Behavioural Conditioning as the Mediator of Placebo Responses in the Immune System," *Philosophical Transactions of the Royal Society of London B: Biological Sciences* 366 (2011): 1799–1807; R Ader, "Conditioned Immunomodulation: Research Needs and Directions," *Brain, Behavior, and Immunity* 17 (2003): S51–S57; MU Goebel, AE Trebst, J Steiner, YF Xie, MS Exton, S Frede, AE Canbay, MC Michel, U Heemann, and M Schedlowski, "Behavioral Conditioning of Immunosuppression Is Possible in Humans," *FASEB Journal* 16 (2002): 1869–73; F Benedetti, A Pollo, L Lopiano, M Lanotte, S Vighetti, and I Rainero, "Conscious Expectation and Unconscious Conditioning in Analgesic, Motor and Hormonal Placebo/Nocebo Responses," *Journal of Neuroscience* 23 (2003): 4315–23; K Meissner, "Effects of Placebo Interventions on Gastric Motility and General Autonomic Activity," *Journal of Psychosomatic Research* 66 (2009): 391–98; SA Isenberg, PM Lehrer, and S Hochron, "The Effects of Suggestion and Emotional Arousal on Pulmonary Function in Asthma: A Review and a Hypothesis Regarding Vagal Mediation," *Psychosomatic Medicine* 54 (1992): 192–216; ME Kemeny, LJ Rosenwasser, RA Panettieri, RM Rose, SM Berg-Smith, and Kline, "Placebo Response in Asthma: A Robust and Objective Phenomenon. *Journal of Allergy and Clinical Immunology* 119 (2007): 1375–81; F Benedetti, M Amanzio, S Baldi, C Casadio, and G Maggi G, "Inducing Placebo Respiratory Depressant Responses in Humans via Opioid Receptors," *European Journal of Neuroscience* 11 (1999): 625–31; A Pollo, S Vighetti, I Rainero I, and F Benedetti, "Placebo Analgesia and the Heart," *Pain* 102(2003): 125–33; K Meissner, "The Placebo Effect and the Autonomic Nervous System: Evidence for an Intimate Relationship," *Philosophical Transaction of the Royal Society of London B: Biological Science* 366: (2011) 1808–1817;

K Meissner and D Ziep, "Organ-Specificity of Placebo Effects on Blood Pressure," *Autonomic Neuroscience* 164: (2011) 62–66; J Ronel, J Mehilli, K-H Ladwig, H Blättler, N Oversohl, RA Byrne, A Bauer, S Schneider, K Linde, P Henningsen, C Lahmann, M Noll-Hussong, and K Meissner, "Effects of Verbal Suggestion on Coronary Arteries: Results of a Randomized Controlled Experimental Investigation During Coronary Angiography," *American Heart Journal* 162 (2011): 507–511

62 F Benedetti, L Colloca, E Torre, M Lanotte, A Melcarne, M Pesare, B Bergamasco, and L Lopiano L, "Placebo-Responsive Parkinson Patients Show Decreased Activity in Single Neurons of Subthalamic Nucleus," *Nature Neuroscience* 7 (2004): 587–88.

63 P Petrovic, E Kalso, KM Petersson, and M Ingvar Placebo and Opioid Analgesia: Imaging a Shared Neuronal Network," *Science* 295 (2002): 1737–40; TD Wager and Barrett L Feldman, "From Affect to Control: Functional Specialization of the Insula in Motivation and Regulation," *PsycExtra* (2004); JK Zubieta, JA Bueller, LR Jackson, DJ Scott, Y Xu, RA Koeppe, and CS Stohler, "Placebo Effects Mediated by Endogenous Opioid Neurotransmission and M-Opioid Receptors," *Journal of Neuroscience* 25 (2005): 7754–62; Zubieta et al. "Placebo Effects Mediated," 7754–62; TD Wager, DJ Scott, and JK Zubieta JK "Placebo Effects on Human Mu-Opioid Activity during Pain," *Proceedings of the National Academy of Science of the United States of America* 104 (2007): 11056–61; F Eippert, U Bingel, ED Schoell, J Yacubian, R Klinger, J Lorenz, and C Büchel, "Activation of the Opioidergic Descending Pain Control System Underlies Placebo Analgesia," *Neuron* 63 (2009): 533–43; A Watson, W El-Deredy, GD Iannetti, D Lloyd, I Tracey, BA Vogt, V Nadeau, and AKP Jones AKP, "Placebo Conditioning and Placebo Analgesia Modulate a Common Brain Network during Pain Anticipation and Perception," *Pain* 145 (2009): 24–30; F Lui, L Colloca, D Duzzi, D Anchisi, F Benedetti, and CA Porro, "Neural Bases of Conditioned Placebo Analgesia," *Pain* 151 (2010): 816–824; TD Wager, LY Atlas, LA Leotti, and JK Rilling, "Predicting Individual Differences in Placebo Analgesia: Contributions of Brain Activity during Anticipation and Pain Experience," *Journal of Neuroscience* 31 (2011): 439–452; TD Wager TD and H Fields, in *Wall and Melzack's Textbook of Pain*, Placebo analgesia, eds. (2011); SB McMahon and M Koltzenburg (Churchill Livingstone, Oxford) in press, Ed 6.; P Krummenacher, V Candia, G Folkers, M Schedlowski, and G Schönbächler, "Prefrontal Cortex Modulates Placebo Analgesia" *Pain* 148 (2010): 368–374.

64 J Borg, O Melander, L Johansson, K Uvnäs-Moberg, JF Rehfeld, and B Ohlsson, "Gastroparesis Is Associated with Oxytocin Deficiency, Oesophageal Dysmotility with Hypercckemia, and Autonomic Neuropathy with Hypergastrinemia," *BMC Gastroenterol* 9 (February 25, 2009):17, doi: 10.1186/1471-230X-9-17; MG Cattaneo, G Lucci, and LM Vicentini, "Oxytocin Stimulates In Vitro Angiogenesis via a Pyk-2/Src-Dependent Mechanism," *Experimental Cell Research 315*, no. 18 (November 1, 2009): 3210–19, doi: 10.1016/j.yexcr.2009.06.022. Epub June 27, 2009; A Szeto, DA Nation, AJ Mendez, J Dominguez-Bendala, LG Brooks, N Schneiderman, and PM McCabe, "Oxytocin Attenuates NADPH-Dependent ç and IL-6 secretion in Macrophages and Vascular Cells," *American Journal of Physiology-Endocrinology Metabolism* 295, no. 6 (December 2008): E1495–501, doi: 10.1152/ajpendo.90718.2008. Epub October 21, 2008; HJ Monstein, N Grahn, M Truedsson, and B Ohlsson, "Oxytocin and Oxytocin-Receptor mRNA Expression in the Human Gastrointestinal Tract: A Polymerase Chain Reaction Study," *Regularity Peptides* 119, no. 1–2 (June 15, 2004): 39–44.

65 T Maruta, RC Colligan, M Malinchoc, and KP Offord, "Optimists vs. Pessimists: Survival Rate among Medical Patients over a 30-Year Period," *Mayo Clinic Proceedings* 75, no. 2 (February 2000): 140–43.

66 T Maruta, RC Colligan, M Malinchoc, and KP Offord, "Optimism-Pessimism Assessed in the 1960s and Self-Reported Health Status 30 Years Later," *Mayo Clinic Proceedings* 77, no. 8 (August 2002): 748–53.

67 AL Geers, SG Helfer, K Kosbab, PE Weiland, and SJ Landry, "Reconsidering the Role of Personality in Placebo Effects: Dispositional Optimism, Situational Expectations, and the Placebo Response. *Journal of Psychosomatic Research* 58 (2005): 121–27; AL Geers, JA Wellman, SL Fowler, SG Helfer, and CR France, "Dispositional Optimism Predicts Placebo Analgesia," *Journal of Pain* 11 (2010): 1165–71; DL Morton, CA Brown, A Watson, W El-Deredy, and AKP Jones, "Cognitive Changes as a Result of a Single Exposure to Placebo," *Neuropsychologia* 48 (2010): 1958–64.

68 BR Levy, MD Slade, SR Kunkel, and SV Kasl, "Longevity Increased by Positive Self-Perceptions of Aging," *J Personality and Social Psychology* 83, no. 2 (August 2002): 261–70.

69 BE Kok, KA Coffey, MA Cohn, LI Catalino, T Vacharkulksemsuk, SB Algoe, M Brantley, and BL Fredrickson, "How Positive Emotions Build Physical Health: Perceived Positive Social Connections Account for the Upward Spiral between Positive Emotions and Vagal Tone," *Psychological*

Science 24, no. 7 (July 1, 2013): 1123–32, doi: 10.1177/0956797612470827, Epub May 6 2013.

70 I Kirsch and G Sapirstein, "Listening to Prozac but Hearing Placebo: A Meta-Analysis of Antidepressant Medication," *Prevention and Treatment* I, article 0002a (1998), http://journals.apa.org/prevention/volume1/pre0010002a.html.

71 I Kirsch, BJ Deacon, TB Huedo-Medina, A Scoboria, TJ Moore, and BT Johnson, "Initial Severity and Antidepressant Benefits: A Meta-Analysis of Data Submitted to the Food and Drug Administration," *PLOS Medicine* 5, no. 2 (February 2008): e45.

72 RJ DeRubeis, LA Gelfand, TZ Tang, and AD Simons, "Medications versus Cognitive Behavior Therapy for Severely Depressed Outpatients: Mega-Analysis of Four Randomized Comparisons," *American Journal of Psychiatry* 156 (1999): 1007–1013; RJ DeRubeis, SD Hollon, JD Amsterdam, and RC Shelton RC, "Cognitive Therapy vs Medications in the Treatment of Moderate to Severe Depression," *Archives of General Psychiatry* 62 (2005): 409–416; M Enserink, "Can the Placebo be the Cure?" *Science* 284 (1999): 238–40; A Khan, HA Warner, and WA Brown WA, "Symptom Reduction and Suicide Risk in Patients Treated with Placebo in Antidepressant Clinical Trials: An Analysis of the FDA Database," *Archives of General Psychiatry* 57 (2000): 311–17; FM Quitkin and DF Klein, "What Conditions are Necessary to Assess Anti-Depressant Efficacy?" *Archives of General Psychiatry* 57 (2000): 323–24; FRM Quitkin, JG Rabkin, J Gerald, JM Davis, and DF Klein, "Validity of Clinical Trails of Antidepressants, *American Journal of Psychiatry* 157 (2000): 327–37; BT Walsh, SN Seidman, R Sysko, and M Gould, "Placebo Response in Studies of Major Depression: Variable, Substantial, and Growing," *JAMA* 287 (2002): 1840–47; F Koerselman, DM Laman, H van Duijn, MA van Duijn, and MA Willems, "A 3-Month, Follow-Up, Randomized, Placebo-Controlled Study Of Repetitive Transcranial Magnetic Stimulation in Depression," *Journal of Clinical Psychiatry* 65 (2004): 1323–28.

73 Fabrizio Benedetti, Helen S. Mayberg, Tor D. Wager, Christian S. Stohler, and Jon-Kar Zubieta, "Neurobiological Mechanisms of the Placebo Effect," *The Journal of Neuroscience* 25, no. 45 (November 9, 2005): 10390–402, doi: 10.1523/JNEUROSCI.3458-05.2005.

74 A Khan et al., "Symptom Reduction and Suicide Risk," 311–17; G Andrews, "Placebo Response in Depression: Bane of Research, Boon to

Therapy," *British Journal of Psychiatry* 178 (2001): 192–94; BT Walsh et al., "Placebo Response in Studies of Major Depression," 1840–47.

75 L Colloca and F Benedetti F, "Placebo Analgesia Induced by Social Observational Learning," *Pain* 144 (2009): 28–34.

76 TJ Kaptchuk, E Friedlander, JM Kelley, MN Sanchez, E Kokkotou, JP Singer, M Kowalczykowski, FG Miller, I Kirsch, and AJ Lembo, "Placebos without Deception: A Randomized Controlled Trial in Irritable Bowel Syndrome," *PLOS One.* 5, no. 12 (December 2010): e15591, doi: 10.1371/journal.pone.0015591.

77 L Colloca, L Lopiano, M Lanotte, and F Benedetti, "Overt versus Covert Treatment for Pain, Anxiety and Parkinson's Disease," *Lancet Neurology* 3 (2004): 679–84.

78 ND Volkow, G-J Wang, Y Ma, JS Fowler, W Zhu, L Maynard, F Telang, P Vaska, Y-S Ding, C Wong, and JM Swanson, "Expectation Enhances the Regional Brain Metabolic and the Reinforcing Effects of Stimulants in Cocaine Abusers," *Journal of Neuroscience* 23 (2003): 11461–68.

79 U Bingel, V Wanigasekera, K Wiech, R Ni Mhuircheartaigh, MC Lee, M Ploner, and I Tracey, "The Effect of Treatment Expectation on Drug Efficacy: Imaging the Analgesic Benefit of the Opioid Remifentanil," *Science Translational Medicine* (2011): 16;3(70).

80 RC Pogge, "The Toxic Placebo. Part I. Side and Toxic Effects Reported during the Administration of Placebo Medicine," *Medical Times* 91: 773–778, 1963.

81 Y Ikemi and S Nakagawa, "A Psychosomatic Study of Contagious Dermatitis," *Kyushu Journal of Medical Science* 13 (1962):335–50.

82 F Benedetti, M Lanotte, L Lopiano, and L Colloca L, "When Words Are Painful: Unraveling the Mechanisms of the Nocebo Effect," *Neuroscience* 147 (2007): 260–71; L Colloca and F Benedetti, "Nocebo Hyperalgesia: How Anxiety Is Turned into Pain," *Current Opinion in Anaesthesiology* 20 (2007): 435–39.

83 Dennis T. Jaffe, PhD, *Healing from Within* (New York: Simon & Schuster, 1986).

84 Rollin McCraty, Mike Atkinson, and Dana Tomasino, "Modulation of DNA Conformation by Heart-Focused Intention," HeartMath Research Center, Institute of HeartMath, Boulder Creek, CA, publication no. 03-008 (2003).

85 DO Hebb, *The Organization of Behaviour: A Neuropsychological Theory* (Mahwah, NJ: Lawrence Erlbaum Associates, Inc., 2002).

86 A Pascual-Leone et al., "Modulation of Muscle Responses Evoked by Transcranial Magnetic Stimulation during the Acquisition of New Fine Motor Skills," *Journal of Neurophysiology* 74, no. 3 (1995): 1037–45.

87 Kazuo Murakami, PhD, *The Divine Code of Life: Awaken Your Genes and Discover Hidden Talents* (Hillsboro, OR: Beyond Words Publishing, 2006).

88 Joe Dispenza, *Evolve Your Brain: The Science of Changing Your Mind* (Deerfield Beach, FL: Health Communications, Inc., 2007).

89 LC Almekinder. "Anti-Inflammatory Treatment of Muscular Injuries in Sport: An Update of Recent Studies," *Sport Medicine* 28 (1999): 383–88.

90 B Hamilton and M Robinson, "Medical Management of Hamstring Injuries," *Aspetar Sports Medicine Journal* (October 2013) 462–66.

91 "Evidence-Based Medicine: A New Approach to Teaching the Practice of Medicine," *JAMA: Journal of the American Medical Association* (1992).

92 Cochrane, "Effectiveness and Efficiency," 1972.

93 I Baruss, *Authentic Knowing* (Purdue University Press, 1996).

94 *BMJ* 327 (December 18, 2003), doi: http://dx.doi.org/10.1136/bmj.327.7429.1459.

95 G Bakris, M Dickholtz Sr., PM Meyer, G Kravitz, E Avery, M Miller, J Brown, C Woodfield, and B Bell, "Atlas Vertebra Realignment and Achievement of Arterial Pressure Goal in Hypertensive Patients: A Pilot Study," *Journal of Human Hypertension* 21, no. 5 (2007 May): 347–52, Epub March 2 2007.

96 Altmann & Bland, 1995

97 Sacket DL, Straus SE, Richardson WS, et al. "Evidence-based medicine: how to practice and teach EBM. 2nd ed. Edinburgh: Churchill Livingstone, 2000.

98 D. D. Palmer (founder of chiropractic), *The Science, Art and Philosophy of Chiropractic: The Chiropractor's Adjuster* (Davenport, IA: Portland Printing House, The Palmer College of Chiropractic, 1910).

99 Stephenson RW. "Chiropractic Textbook";1927.

100 Palmer, *Science, Art and Philosophy.*

101 *Aphorisms of Dr. Charles Horace Mayo and Dr. William James Mayo* (Springfield, IL: Charles C. Thomas Publisher, 1951).

102 Ola Dale, Petter C Borchgrevink, Olav Fredheim, Milada Mahic, Pål Romundstad, and Svetlana Skurtveit, "Prevalence of Use of Non-Prescription Analgesics in the Norwegian HUNT3 Population: Impact of Gender, Age, Exercise And Prescription of Opioids," *BMC Public Health* 15 (2015): 461 (May 2, 2015, open access).

103 Philip Cohen, Philip, "Mental Gymnastics Increase Biceps Strength," *New Scientist* (November 21, 2001).

104 G Yue and K. J. Cole, "Strength Increase from the Motor Program: Comparison of Training with Maximal Voluntary and Imagined Muscle Contractions," *Journal of Neurophysiology* 67, no. 5 (1992): 1114–23.

105 J. H. Tilden, MD, *Impaired Health*, 3rd ed. (Mokelumne Hill, California: Health Research, 1921, 1960).

106 Dennis T. Jaffe, PhD, *Healing from Within*, (New York: Simon & Schuster, Inc., 1986).

107 Robert S. Mendelsohn, MD, *Male Practice* (Chicago: Contemporary Books, Inc., 1982), 11.

108 M McCoy, "Evaluation of a Standardized Wellness Protocol to Improve Anthropometric and Physiologic Function and to Reduce Health Risk Factors: A Retrospective Analysis of Outcome," *Journal of Alternative and Complementary Medicine* 17, no. 1 (January 2011): 39–44, doi: 10.1089/acm.2010.0113, Epub January 3, 2011.

109 Palmer, *Science, Art and Philosophy*.

110 Fratello et al., "Modulation of Corticospinal Excitability," 2667–74; J Liepert, H Bauder, HR Wolfgang, WH Miltner, E Taub, and C Weiller, "Treatment- Induced Cortical Reorganization after Stroke in Humans," *Stroke* 31, no. 6 (June 2000): 1210–16; Sessle et al., "Properties and Plasticity Induced," 259–66; Tinazzi et al., "Plastic Interactions," 769–776; Weiss et al., "Rapid Functional Plasticity," 3413–3423; Sanes and Donoghue, "Plasticity and Primary Motor Cortex," 393–415; Tye et al., "Motor Cortex Plasticity Induced," 259–66; Kalin-Lang et al., "Role of Voluntary Drive," 1099–1103.

111 H Haavik and Murphy B, "The Role of Spinal Manipulation in Addressing Disordered Sensorimotor Integration and Altered Motor Control. *Journal of Electromyography and Kinesiology* 22, no. 5 (October 2012): 768–76; H Haavik, H Taylor, K Holt, and B Murphy, "Exploring the Neuromodulatory Effects of the Vertebral Subluxation and Chiropractic Care," *Chiropractic Journal of Australia*; H Haavik, H Taylor, and B Murphy, "Cervical Spine Manipulation Alters Sensorimotor Integration: A Somatosensory Evoked Potential Study," *Clinical Neurophysiology* 118, no. 2 (2007): 391–402.

112 H Haavik, H Taylor, and B Murphy, "Transient Modulation of Intracortical Inhibition Following Spinal Manipulation," *Chiropractic Journal of Australia* 37 (2007): 106–16; H Haavik and B Murphy, "Altered Sensorimotor Integration with Cervical Spine Manipulation," *Journal of*

Manipulative and Physiological Therapeutics 31, no. 2 (2008): 115–26; I Niazi, K Turker, S Flavel, M Kingett, J Duehr, and H Haavik, "Increased Cortical Drive and Altered Net Excitability and Low-Threshold Motor Unit Levels to the Lower Limb Following Spinal Manipulation," paper presented at World Federation of Chiropractic's 12th Biennial Congress, April 6–9, 2013, Durban, South Africa.

113 LC Boyd-Clark, CA Briggs, and Galea MP. "Muscle Spindel Distribution, Morphology, and Density in Longus Colli and Multifidus Muscles of the Cervical Spine," *SPINE* 27, no. 2 (2002): 694–701.

114 V Kulkarni, MJ Chandy, and KS Babu, "Quantitative Study of Muscle Spindles in Suboccipital Muscles On Human Foetuses," *Neurol India* 49 (2001): 355–59.

115 S Cooper and P Daniel, "Muscle Spindles in Man: Their Morphology in the Lumbricals and the Deep Muscles of the Neck," *Brain* 86 (1963): 563–94.

116 Amonoo-Kuofi, "The Density of Muscle Spindles in the Medial, Intermediate and Lateral Columns of Human Intrinsic Postvertebral Muscles." *Journal of Anatomy* 136, no. 3 (1983): 509–519.

117 Frederick H. Barge, DC, PhC, *One Cause One Cure*, 1990.

118 W Herzhog, "Mechanical, Physiologic and Neuromuscular Considerations of Chiropractic Treatment" in DJ Lawrence, JD Cassidy, M McGregor, WC Meeker, and HT Vernon, eds., *Advances in Chiropractic* Vol. 3 (New York: Mosby-Year Book, 1996), 269–85.

119 W Herzog W, D Scheele, and PJ Conway, "Electromyographic Responses of Back and Limb Muscles Associated with Spinal Manipulative Therapy," *Spine* 24, no. 2 (1999): 146–53.

120 Haavik and Murphy, "Spinal Manipulation in Disordered Sensorimotor Integration," 768–76; Haavik et al., "Exploring the Neuromodulatory Effects"; Haavik et al., "Cervical Spine Manipulation Alters Sensorimotor Integration," 391–402; H Haavik, H Taylor, and B Murphy, "Altered Central Integration of Dual Somatosensory Input Observed Following Motor Training: A Crossover Study," *Journal of Manipulative & Physiological Therapeutics* 33, no. 3 (2010): 178–88.

121 H Haavik and B Murphy, "Subclinical Neck Pain and the Effects of Cervical Manipulation on Elbow Joint Sense," *Journal of Manipulative & Physiological Therapeutics* 34 (2011): 88–97; K Holt, *Effectiveness of Chiropractic Care in Improving Sensorimotor Function associated with Fall Risk in Older People* (Auckland, New Zealand: Department of Population Health, University of Auckland, 2013).

122 P Hodges and C Richardson, "Altered Trunk Muscle Recruitment in People with Low Back Pain with Upper Limb Movement at Different Speeds," *Archives of Physical Medicine and Rehabilitation* 80 (1999): 1005–1012; A Radebold, J Cholewicki, GK Polzhofer, and HS Greene, "Impaired Postural Control of the Lumbar Spine is Associated with Delayed Muscle Response Times in Patients with Chronic Idiopathic Low Back Pain," *Spine* 26, no. 7 (2001): 724–30; JH Van Dieen, LP Selen, and J Cholewicki, "Trunk Muscle Activation in Low-Back Pain Patients: An Analysis of the Literature," *Journal of Electromyography and Kinesiology* 13, no. 4 (2003): 333–51; J Cholewicki, S Silfies, R Shah, et al., "Delayed Muscle Trunk Reflex Responses Increase the Risk of Low Back Injuries," *Spine* 30, no. 23 (2005): 2614–20 (Philadelphia, PA, 1976).

123 P Marshall and B Murphy, "The Effect of Sacroiliac Joint Manipulation on Feed-Forward Activation Times of the Deep Abdominal Musculature," *Journal of Manipulative and Physiological Therapeutics* 29, no. 3(2006): 196–202.

124 SM Cowan SM and KL Benell, PW Hodges, KM Crossley, and J McConnell, "Simultaneous Feedforward Recruitment of the Vasti in Untrained Postural Tasks Can Be Restored by Physical Therapy," *Journal of Orthopaedic Research* 21, no. 3 (2003): 553–58; D Falla, "Unraveling the Complexity of Muscle Impairment in Chronic Neck Pain," *Manual Therapy* 9, no. 3 (August 2004): 125–33.

125 Haavik and Murphy, "Subclinical Neck Pain," 88–97; Holt, *Chiropractic Care in Improving Sensorimotor Function.*

126 R. A. Coronado, C. W. Gay, J. E. Bialosky, G. D. Carnaby, M. D. Bishop, and S. Z. George, "Changes in Pain Sensitivity Following Spinal Manipulation: A Systematic Review and Meta-Analysis," *Journal of Electromyography Kinesiology* 22, no. 5 (2012), 752–67.

127 W. R. Reed, J. G. Pickar, R. S. Sozio, and C. R. Long, "Effect of Spinal Manipulation Thrust Magnitude on Trunk Mechanical Activation Thresholds of Lateral Thalamic Neurons," *Journal of Manipulative and Physiological Therapeutics* 37, no. 5 (2014), 277–86.

128 P Mohammadian, A Gonsalves, C Tsai, T Hummel, and T Carpenter, "Areas of Capsaicin-Induced Secondary Hyperalgesia and Allodynia Are Reduced by a Single Chiropractic Adjustment: A Preliminary Study," *Journal of Manipulative and Physiological Therapeutic* 27, no. 6 (2004): 381–87.

129 C. W. Gay, M. E. Robinson, S. Z. George, W. M. Perlstein, and M. D. Bishop, "Immediate Changes after Manual Therapy in Resting-State Functional Connectivity as Measured by Functional Magnetic Resonance Imaging in Participants with Induced Low Back Pain," *Journal of Manipulative and Physiological Therapeutics* 37, no. 9 (2014), 614–27.

130 Bakris et al., "Atlas Vertebra Realignment," 347–52.

131 PL Rome, "Neurovertebral Influence upon the Autonomic Nervous System: Some of the Somato-Autonomic Evidence to Date," *Chiropractic Journal of Australia* 39 (2009): 2–17.

132 J Zhang J, D Dean, D Nosco, D Strathopulos, and M Floros, "Effect of Chiropractic Care on Heart Rate Variability and Pain in a Multisite Clinical Study," *Journal of Manipulative Physiological Therapeutics* 29, no. 4 (May 2006): 267–74.

133 M Sterling, G Jull, B Vicenzino, RDY J Kena, and R Darnell, "Development of Motor System Dysfunction Following Constantly Whiplash Injury, *Pain* 103, no. 1–2 (2003): 65–73; G Jull, P Trott, H Potter, et al., "Randomized Controlled Trial of Exercise and Manipulative Therapy for Cervicogenic Headache," *Spine* 27, no. 17 (September 2002): 1835–43.

134 S Brumagne, P Cordo, R Lysens, S Verschuren, and S Swinna, "The Role of Paraspinal Muscle Spindles in Lumbosacral Position Sensing in Individuals with and without Low Back Pain," *Spine* 25, no. 8 (2000): 989–94; P Michaelson, M Michaelson, S Jarić, ML Latasha, P Sjolander, and M Djupsjobacka, "Vertical Posture and Head Stability in Patients with Chronic Neck Pain," *Journal of Rehabilitation Medicine* 25, no. 23 (2003): 229–35.

135 SM Hannon, "Objective Physiologic Changes and Associated Health Benefits of Chiropractic Adjustments in Asymptomatic Subjects: A Review of the Literature," *Journal of Vertebral Subluxation Research* (April 26, 2004), 1–9.

136 L Goldstein and H Makofsky. "TMD / Facial Pain and Forward Head Posture," *Practical Pain Management* 5, no. 5 (July/August 2005), 36–39.

137 Carney et al., "Power Posing, Brief Non-Verbal Displays Affect Neuroendocrine Levels and Risk Tolerance," *Psychological Science* 21, no. 10 (2010): 1363–68.

138 S Arnette and T Pettijohn, "The Effects of Posture on Self-Perceived Leadership," *International Journal of Business and Social Science* 3, no. 14 (2012), 8–13.

139 P Brinol et al., "Body Posture Effects on Self-Evaluation: A Self-Validation Approach," *European Journal of Self Psychology* 39 (2009): 1053–64.

140 A Apkarian et al., "Chronic Back Pain is Associated with Decreased Prefrontal and Thalamic Gray Matter Density," *Journal of Neuroscience* 24, no. 46 (2004).

141 Cailliet and L Gross, *Rejuvenation Strategy* (New York: Doubleday Co., 1987).

142 J Deuchars and I Edwards, "Bad Posture Could Raise Your Blood Pressure," *Journal of Neuroscience* (2007), 0638–07.

143 E Lopes et al., "Assessment of Muscle Shortening and Static Posture in Children with Persistent Asthma, *European Journal of Pediatrics* 166, no. 7 (2006), 715–21.

144 D Kado, M Huang, E Barrett-Connor, and G Greendale, "Hyperkyphotic Posture and Poor Physical Functional Ability in Older Community-Dwelling Men and Women: The Rancho Bernardo Study," *Journals of Gerontology: Biological Sciences* 60, no. 5 (2005), 633–37.

145 D Kado et al., Hyperkyphosis Predict Mortality Independent of Vertebral Osteoporosis in Older Women," *Annals of Internal Medicine* 150 (2009): 681–87.

146 S Wannamethee, A Shaper, L Lennon, and P Whincup, "Height Loss in Older Men: Associations with Total Mortality and Incidence of Cardiovascular Disease," *Archives of Internal Medicine* 166, no. 22 (2006) 2546–52.

147 Kado et al., "Hyperkyphotic Posture and Risk of Injurious Falls," 652–57.

148 O'Sullivan et al., "Posture and Low Back Pain," *Spine* 27 (2002): 1238–44.

149 S Jones et al., "Individuals with Non-Specific Low Back Pain Use a Trunk Stiffening Strategy to Maintain Upright Posture," *Journal of Electromyography and Kinesiology* 22, no. 1(2011): 13–20.